Craniofacial Surgery - Recent Advances, New Perspectives and Applications

Edited by Belma Işik Aslan and Serhat Şibar

Published in London, United Kingdom

Craniofacial Surgery - Recent Advances, New Perspectives and Applications
http://dx.doi.org/10.5772/intechopen.102235
Edited by Belma Işik Aslan and Serhat Şibar

Contributors
Belma Işik Aslan, Şeyma Akçay Gülşen, Şadiye Bacık Tırank, Mohammad Zeinalddin, Nikita Khilion, Amine Fattal, Simone La Padula, Rosita Pensato, Rebecca Sabban, Francesco D'Andrea, Edoardo Coiante, Giovanni Roccaro, Mounia SidAhmed-Mezi, Jean Paul Meningaud, Barbara Hersant, Surya Sudhakar V. Goparaju, Naida Hadziabdic, Robert Pellecchia, Benjamin Richardson, Anirudh Nair, Farajollah Soleimanzadeh, Kambiz Vatandoost, Gunanand D. Persaud III

First published in London, United Kingdom, 2023 by IntechOpen
IntechOpen is the global imprint of INTECHOPEN LIMITED, registered in England and Wales, registration number: 11086078, 5 Princes Gate Court, London, SW7 2QJ, United Kingdom

British Library Cataloguing-in-Publication Data
A catalogue record for this book is available from the British Library

Additional hard and PDF copies can be obtained from orders@intechopen.com

Craniofacial Surgery - Recent Advances, New Perspectives and Applications
Edited by Belma Işik Aslan and Serhat Şibar
p. cm.
Print ISBN 978-1-80355-468-6
Online ISBN 978-1-80355-469-3
eBook (PDF) ISBN 978-1-80355-470-9

Meet the editors

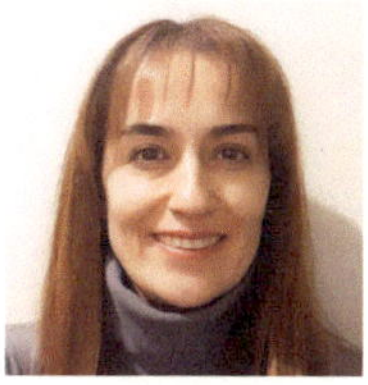

Prof. Dr. Belma Işik Aslan obtained a Ph.D. in Orthodontic Education from Gazi University, Turkey, in 2005. In 2006, she visited the Providence Hospital Institute for Craniofacial and Reconstructive Surgery, USA, for three months as an observer. She was appointed as an associate professor in 2014 and as a professor in 2021. She still works as an instructor at the same faculty. She has thirty-six journal articles, one book, twelve book chapters, and forty conference proceedings to her credit. She is a member of the Turkish Orthodontic Society and the Turkish Cleft Lip and Palate Society.

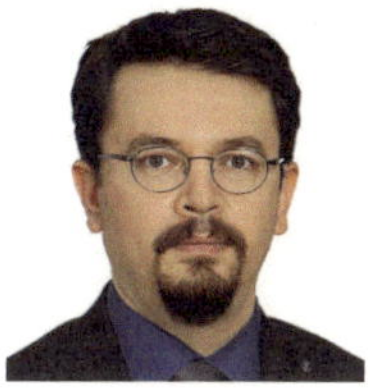

Assoc. Prof. Serhat Şibar completed his plastic surgery residency at Gazi University, Turkey, in 2016. He visited the El Paso Plastic Surgery in Texas, USA, for two months as an observer. He has been working as an academic staff since 2018. He has thirty-three journal articles, one book, six book chapters, and seventy conference proceedings to his credit. He is a member of the Turkish Society of Plastic Surgery, Turkish Society of Reconstructive Microsurgery, Turkish Society of Aesthetic Plastic Surgery, and International Society of Aesthetic and Plastic Surgery.

Contents

Preface

This book provides information on current advances, new perspectives, and applications in craniofacial surgery. The topics discussed include regenerative materials in oral surgery, tissue induction in plastic and maxillo-facial surgery, the role of genetics, stem cells, and reconstructive surgery in craniofacial diseases and syndromes, diagnostic and surgical considerations in congenital craniofacial deformities such as cleft lip and palate (CLP) and craniosynostosis, and assessment of psychological functioning in cleft lip palate patients.

Chapter 1, 'Protocols in Presurgical Infant Orthopaedic Treatment—An Evidence Based Review', presents scientific literature on current presurgical infant orthopedics (PSIO) treatment appliances in patients with CLP and analyses the current state of PSIO.

Chapter 2, 'Perspective Chapter: Role of Genetics, Stem Cells in Reconstructive Surgery—Their Perspectives in Craniofacial Diseases and Syndromes', discusses genetic screening and gene therapy in patients with craniofacial malformations as well as the application of stem cells in the reconstruction of the maxillofacial region and treatment of head and neck pathology.

Chapter 3, 'Tissue Induction in Plastic and Maxillo-Facial Surgery' details the various current techniques for tissue regeneration in the field of plastic and maxillo-facial surgery.

Chapter 4, 'PRF and Sticky Bone as Regenerative Materials in Oral Surgery', discusses the preparation of platelet-rich fibrin (PRF) membranes and other platelet concentrates with the sticky bone to facilitate the bone regeneration process.

Chapter 5, 'A Review of Current Surgical Approaches and Diagnostic Features Associated with Craniosynostosis Patients and the Relation to Oral and Maxillofacial Surgery', reviews the current surgical approaches to and diagnostic features of craniosynostosis in relation to oral and maxillofacial surgery.

Chapter 6, 'Assessment of Psychosocial Functioning among Patients with Cleft Lip/Palate and Their Mothers', examines the psychosocial status of both children and adolescents with CLP and their mothers in a large-scale and multidimensional manner.

The book is a useful resource for craniofacial surgeons, orthodontic practitioners, and students in the field.

We would like to thank all the authors and the staff at IntechOpen, especially Author Service Manager Ms. Dolores Kuzelj, for their assistance throughout the publication process. We are also thankful to Prof. Dr. Ayşe Gülşen for her valuable assistance.

Belma Işik Aslan
Gazi University Dentistry Faculty,
Department of Orthodontics,
Ankara, Türkiye

Serhat Şibar
Gazi University Medical Faculty,
Department of Plastic, Reconstructive and Aesthetic Surgery,
Ankara, Türkiye

Chapter 1

Protocols in Presurgical Infant Orthopaedic Treatment—An Evidence Based Review

Nikita Khillon, Amine Fattal and Mohammad Zeinalddin

Abstract

Presurgical infant orthopaedic (PSIO) protocol is applied prior to cleft Lip and/cleft palate surgical intervention to facilitate the repair by restoring the alar base and maintaining the skeletal, soft tissue harmony. The objective of this review is to assess the literature on the presurgical infant orthopaedic protocol most widely used and accepted. Searches were made in PubMed, Cochrane and Google Scholar on cleft lip and/palate. A large number of articles documented approaching PSIO for cleft treatment with the intent to provide a satisfactory treatment for cleft patients, requiring far more than just correctional surgery and its ability to do so is unique. Craniofacial Orthodontists can choose from a wide array of treatment options for their patients and can learn from the outcomes attained by applying a combination of outcomes at various other centers.

Keywords: Systematic review, cleft lip, cleft palate, presurgical, infant orthopaedics, PSIO

1. Introduction

Pre-Surgical Infant Orthopaedic (PSIO) protocol indisputably has a valuable impact in the management of cleft lip and palate infants, showing approximation and alignment of alveolar segments and narrowing the gap between lip components, with the intent of separating oral cavity from nasal and maintaining the tongue position. However, nasal cartilage symmetry and increase in the columella length results remain distinctive [1], with long term benefits still under speculations. Although the popularity of NAM has grown by leaps and bounds in the last one decade, it has become essential to annotate the outcome of both NAM and other PSIO protocols. Studies regarding NAM have been either case studies or single center retrospective comparisons of before-and-after clinical features on small samples with no control non-NAM cases.

2. Discussion

An evidence-based approach to cleft lip and palate management in the last two decades has led many craniofacial orthodontists to show great enthusiasm for presurgical infant orthopaedics (PSIO). Patients with unilateral and bilateral complete cleft lip and/palate demand far more than just correctional surgeries. Any manipulations of the infant's orofacial complex prior to nasal and lip surgical repair is conducted under the aegis of term presurgical infant orthopaedics (PSIO).

An inevitable manifestation of cleft lip and palate remains to be primary nasal deformity, presenting a significant surgical challenge requiring patients to undergo multiple surgical procedures.

Advocates of PSIO have stated, besides improving arch form and facilitating arch closure, its main objective is improving nasal symmetry and lip aesthetics. In order to make cleft lip and/or palate care cardinal for these patients, it's essential to understand these protocols and develop a more centralised approach. The aim of the present review is to provide scientific literature on most current PSIO appliances in patients with CLP and to analyse the current state of PSIO (**Table 1**).

This evidence based review registered at the international prospective register of systematic reviews, PROSPERO, with the following registration number CRD42021280979. The report followed the preferred Reporting items for Evidence based reviews and Meta-Analyses (PRISMA) 2020 edition. Three electronic Databases namely PubMed, Cochrane & Google Scholar Library on Cleft-Lip and/Palate were searched and used in the current study. Studies that were conducted between the years 2011 and 2021 with the primary keywords were searched. We used search strategies involving the MeSH descriptors and 61 studies met the inclusion criteria.

The main descriptors used were as follows:

1. MeSH: "Presurgical infant orthopaedics" OR "pre surgical orthopaedics"OR "infant orthopaedics" AND ("Cleft Palate"[Mesh] OR "Cleft Lip"[Mesh] OR "infant" OR "neonatal" OR "unilateral cleft lip and palate".

1. *Pub-Med*: The searches in this database were made in "Search Details."

2. *Cochrane:* The searches in this database were made in "search History", and the search strategy was assembled in "search for".

3. *Google Scholar:* The searches in this database were made in "Google search".

Timing	Procedure
After 16 weeks of pregnancy	cleft lip diagnosis by ultrasound images(Palate is more difficult to acquire)
Prenatal	Discussion with craniofacial surgeon, consultation with a geneticist/ dysmorphologist
Neonatal	If the child has cleft palate, specialised nipples and bottles are necessary to improve feeding after birth
6-12 months of age	12 weeks of age cleft lip repair; cleft palate one-stage repair with intravelar veloplasty
5 years	secondary rhinoplasty

Table 1.
Treatment modalities in the management of unilateral cleft lip and palate which are often based on chronological age.

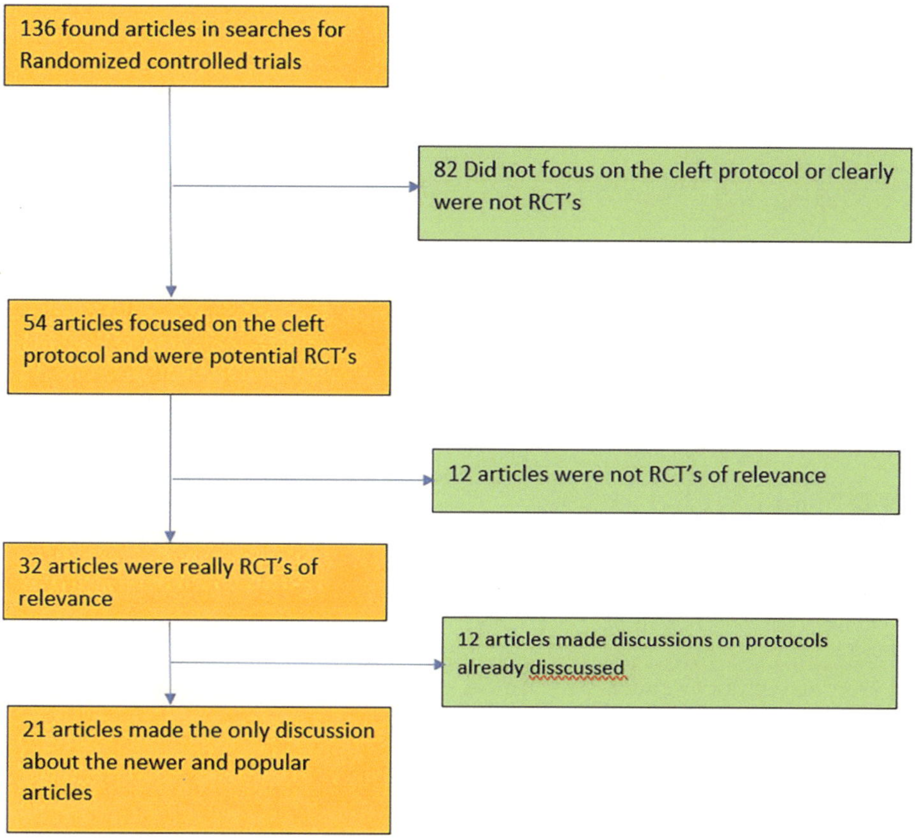

Figure 1.
The flow chart above outlines the selection process of articles.

All abstracts provided by the databases in the searches were collected resulting in a total of 136 articles. From these abstracts, studies that clearly did not include presurgical infant orthopaedics were excluded. After meticulous reading of the full text articles, 21 articles were included for the analysis of the obtained conclusion (**Figure 1**). Further assessment of the literature for inclusion in this review was performed by evaluating the full text based on the selection criteria. Literatures that were not in line with the selection criteria were then excluded from the study. Quality assessment and data synthesis were completed independently by two investigators (NK and AF) and any discrepancies were resolved by consultation with the third author (MZ).

The following inclusion criteria were used for the evidence based review:

1. Study types: RCTs and observational study

2. Study assessed an outcome related to the use of pre-surgical infant orthopaedic

3. Studies done after 2010

4. Studies reported in English language

The protocols enlisted in the 21 articles are as follows:

1. Naso-alveolar Moulding: 7/21 = 33.33%
2. Modified Latham Appliance: 2/21 = 9.52%
3. Lip Taping: 4/21 = 19.04%
4. McNiel: 1/21 = 4.76%
5. Nasal Elevator Device- Dyna Cleft: 1/21 = 4.76%
6. SAC-PP-MR Technique: 1/21 = 4.76%
7. Aligner NAM: 1/21 = 4.76%
8. 3-D Vomer Plate: 2/21 = 9.52%
9. Lip taping w/prefabricated nasal stent: 1/21 = 4.76%
10. Vacuum formed NAM: 1/21 = 4.76%

In order to conduct a successful clinical practice with PSIO protocols, the systematic reviews and RCTs are considered the most appropriate evidence. The main search engine proposed by World Health Organisation i.e. PubMed and Cochrane Library, along with google scholar were used to find the RCTs to formulate a study for evidence based medicine. A total of 136 articles were found, and we reached 21 articles that proposed PSIO protocols on cleft patients.

PSIO came into existence with McNiel in 1950 using buccal plates to manipulate the alveolar segments. Beginning with Grayson and Colleagues [2] in 1993, has inspired many orthodontists over the last few decades to develop a protocol that not only shapes the nasal cartilage, but also mould's the alveolar process. Two of the most favoured PSIO protocols employed are Nasoalveolar moulding and Latham-Millard technique [3] with the later potentiating a successful GPP and obligating nasolabial fistula prior to secondary bone graft [4], while the former aims at reducing the severity of cleft defect in both UCLP and BCLP infants [2]. In UCLP infants the cleft defect between the alveolar segments is approximated, the lip elements are brought close together and the deviated columella is repositioned. For BCLP infants, the Grayson NAM technique successfully retracts the Premaxilla and the alveolar segments are widened for alignment. The columella is elongated non-surgically [2]. The direct benefit of using the Latham device as part of pre-surgical infant dentofacial orthopaedic is ease of gingivoperiosteoplasty. Millards, an acclaimed plastic surgeon, modified the Latham's fixed appliance such that it amalgamated with his surgical protocol reporting a significantly reduced number of fistulas post-operative [5]. However, the Latham dento-maxillary orthopaedic appliance used screws to approximate the alveolar segments in unilateral complete cleft patients. A "Modified Latham "appliance designed by Stephen Ruso and Ernest Ruas at John Hopkins Hospital, Florida claims that the use of elastic power chain instead of screws to approximate the alveolar segments reduces the treatment time to 2 weeks [6].

Lip tapping alone has been labelled as a tyrannised PSIO protocol in spite of it being a simple and inexpensive procedure, which is even more pressing when dealing with a lifelong condition such as cleft lip and palate. The dearth of impression making

Experimental group	Conclusion	Explanation for conclusion
Naso-Alveolar Moulding (NAM)	NAM helps to approximate the segments of cleft maxilla and reduce inter-segment space [2]	For Unilateral cleft cases the NAM Device helps to approximate the greater and lesser segment, simultaneous elevating lateral cartilage and straightening the deviated columella [2]
Modified Latham Appliance	Shorter treatment duration compared to traditional Latham appliance and NAM, making operative placement at an older age feasible [6]	The power chain provides a continuous force application on the palatal segments, bringing the two together in a span of 2 weeks of active therapy without impacting the future growth of facial sutures [6]
Lip taping	Lip taping alone can change the maxillary arch dimensions before surgical lip repair in UCLP infants; A simple and inexpensive type of PSIO [7]	Eliminated the need to make an impression, allowing the treatment to start early and making it inexpensive with a significant change in maxillary arch dimensions
Muscle activated NAM	Helps better alveolar position along with improvement in nasal symmetry, alignment of nasal septum and nasal tip projection [19]	The Device guides the placement of tongue tip thereby preventing the cleft widening effect of tongue allowing the facial musculature movements to act as a guide
Nasal Elevator Device—Dyna Cleft	Significantly reduce the cleft width and improve the nasal asymmetry	The device acts indirectly on the cleft alveolar segments with force vector generated from traction of lip muscles, keeping the nostril airway less restricted and overall technique being less invasive. It is less expensive and easier for parents to manage
Aligner -NAM	Significant increase in the columella length with near-complete approximation of maxillary alveolar segment [20]	Intraoral scanner for recording intraoral impressions is less hazardous and more accurate. Downside of acrylic plate such as ulceration is eliminated [20]
SAC-PP-MR Technique	A modified, economical, comparatively easier and faster technique reducing the defect to zero [12]	A passive appliance stimulates the involved tissues during physiological functions like swallowing and feeding resulting in overcorrection of alar cartilage; the technique derives its basis from functional matrix theory
Latham appliance	Significant reduction in alveolar cleft width allowing for minimal-dissection gingivoperiosteoplasty [5]	Achieved favourable nasolabial aesthetics with midface growth sometimes affected (GOSLON Score 4 or 5) making orthognathic surgery inevitable
Vacuum formed NAM	Significantly reduced alveolar and palatal cleft width along with reduction in midline deviation [21, 22]	A sequential appliance fabrication eliminates the burden of presurgical therapy [21, 22]
Surgical Nasoalveolar moulding	Pre-surgical Naso-Alveolar Moulding followed by primary surgical repair still lacks sufficient scientific evidence when compared to primary cheilorhinoplasty in closing the alveolar gap and improving nasal appearance, therefore NAM is still not considered gold standard [23]	Primary nasal and palatal repair surgery in unilateral cleft lip palate patients, based on a literature review [23]

Table 2.
Conclusion of articles that used various presurgical infant orthopaedic (PSIO) techniques.

and appliance fabrication permits the early start of treatment exhibiting good maxillary arch dimensions and lip approximation [7].

Inspired by the technique employed by Berggren and Berggren et al., in 2002 a simple nasal elevator composed of plastic, with an elastic band pasted on the forehead was used to approximate the cleft edges [8]. A new and simpler way of providing PSIO gave rise to Dynacleft, where the maxillary segments are approximated indirectly aided by force factors coming from lip muscle traction [9]. Due to the dentoalveolar growth and simultaneous cleft reduction, the need for fabricating new plates demands the nasal stents to be re-mounted, adding to the visiting appointments. This leads to a quick-lock system for nasal stent transfer, minimising the wire adaptations. The addition of CAD/CAM technology has not only saved the chair side time, but significantly increased the cleft side nasal height and improved the nasal symmetry [10]. It's use is on ever increasing rise for recording details in cleft-Lip and Palate patients and is relatively less risk averse and more precise when compared to the primitive impression making procedure [11]. A series of case results documenting PSIO cases treated with CAT has opened a window to a new and exciting future [12].

A modified, yet simpler and cheaper technique called "The SAC-PP-MR "technique recently came into existence with the intent to target all, to not only facilitate cheiloplasty and ensure positive aesthetic outcome. It successfully documented reducing the cleft sizc to zcro [12].

Presurgical Infant Orthopaedic Treatment (PSIO) has been accepted and acknowledged into practice by the majority of multidisciplinary cleft teams around the world attributing the cleft defect repair and primary nose surgery [13–15]. An inter center comparison study using Asher-McDade scale demonstrated a significantly favourable outcome in nasolabial appearance scores Vs outcomes resulting from primary surgical repair only [16]. Craniofacial Orthodontists can choose from a wide array of treatment options for their patients and can learn from the outcomes attained by applying a combination of outcomes at various other centers. However, attempts have been made by craniofacial orthodontists to modify PNAM device with the intent to simplify the fabrication and reduce the frequency of recall visits [17]. Distance as a factor has been obsolete from many discussions advocating the use of PSIO or eliciting the need for newer PSIO techniques [18], however it has been revealed to cause a significant difference in the delivery of cleft care (**Table 2**).

3. Conclusion

In Conclusion, Craniofacial Orthodontists can choose from a wide array of treatment options for their patients and can learn from the outcomes attained by applying a combination of outcomes at various other centres. Distance as a factor has been obsolete from many discussions advocating the use of PSIO or eliciting the need for newer PSIO techniques, however it has been revealed to cause a significant difference in the delivery of cleft care.

Authors' contributions

NK—Methodology, data collection, writing manuscript. AF—Methodology, data collection, visualisation, review and editing. MZ—Conceptualisation, data collection, Supervision, Review and editing.

Conflict of interests

The authors declare that there is no conflict of interest.

Author details

Nikita Khillon, Amine Fattal and Mohammad Zeinalddin*
Craniofacial Orthodontics Fellowship, Chang Gung University, Taiwan, China

*Address all correspondence to: dr.mohammad.orthodontics@gmail.com

References

[1] Kapadia H, Olson D. Nasoalveolar moulding for unilateral and bilateral cleft lip repair. Oral and Maxillofacial Surgery Clinics of North America. 2020;**32**:197-204

[2] Grayson BH, Garfinkle JS. Early cleft management: The case for nasoalveolar moulding. American Journal of Orthodontics and Dentofacial Orthopedics. 2014;**145**(2):134-124

[3] Jodeh DS, Ruso S. Clinical outcomes utilizing a "Modified Latham" appliance for presurgical infant orthopedics in patients with unilateral complete cleft lip and palate. The Cleft Palate-Craniofacial Journal. 2019;**56**(7):929-935

[4] Santiago PE, Grayson BH. Reduced need for alveolar bone grafting by presurgical orthopedics and primary gingivoperiosteoplasty. The Cleft Palate-Craniofacial Journal. 1998;**35**(1):77-80

[5] Latham RA. Orthopedic advancement of the cleft maxillary segment: A preliminary report. The Cleft Palate Journal. 1980;**17**(3):227-233

[6] Jodeh DS, Ruso S, Feldman R, Ruas E, Rottgers SA. Clinical outcomes utilizing a "Modified Latham" appliance for presurgical infant orthopedics in patients With Unilateral Complete Cleft Lip and Palate. The Cleft Palate-Craniofacial Journal. 2019;**56**(7):929-935

[7] Ael-G M, Mamdouh A, Salah MM. Is taping alone an efficient Pre-surgical infant orthopedic approach in infants with unilateral cleft lip and palate? A randomized control trial. The cleft-Palate Craniofacial Journal. 2020;**57**(12)

[8] Monasterio L, Mun˜ oz M, Bennun R. Tratamiento Interdisciplinario de la Fisuras Labio-Palatinas. Santiago: Luis Monasterio Aljaro; 2008;**35**(1):133-164

[9] Monasterio L, Ford A. Comparative study of nasoalveolar molding methods: Nasal elevator plus dyna cleft versus NAM-grayson in patients with complete unilateral cleft lip and palate. The Cleft Palate-Craniofacial Journal. 2013;**50**(5):548-554

[10] Grill FD, Lucas M. Ritschl Facilitating CAD/CAM nasoalveolar molding therapy with a novel click-in system for nasal stents ensuring a quick and user-friendly chairside nasal stent exchange. Scientific Report. 2018;**8**:12084. DOI: 10.1038/s41598-018-29960-z

[11] Chalmers EV, McIntyre GT, Wang W, Gillgrass T, Mossey MCB, PA. Intraoral 3D scanning or dental impressions for the assessment of dental arch relationships in cleft care: Which is superior? The Cleft Palate-Craniofacial Journal. 2016;**53**(5):568-577

[12] Elizondo R, Manuel O, Lagravère, Esthela Flores, and Nora Letechipı'a. Presurgical preparation of infants with unilateral cleft lip and palate. The SAC-PP-MR Innovative Technique. 2019;**56**(3):408-414

[13] Bennun R, Perandones C, Sepliarsky V, Chantiri S, Ulfe I, Dogliotti P. Non-surgical correction of nasal deformity in unilateral complete cleft lip: A 6 year follow- up. Plastic Reconstructive Surgery. 1999;**104**:616

[14] Grayson B, Shetya P. Pre-surgical naso-alveolar moulding treatment in CLP patients. Indian Journal of Plastic Surgery Supplement. 2009;**42**(suppl):S56-S61

[15] Liou E, Subramanian M, Chen P, Huang S. The progressive changes of Nasal symmetry and grow after Naso-alveolar moulding: A three year follow-up study. Plastic and Reconstructive Surgery. 2004:114

[16] Peanchitlertkajorn S, Mercado A, Daskalogiannakis J, Hathaway R, Russell K, Semb G, et al. An intercentre comparison of nasolabial appearance including a centre using Naso-Alveolar Moulding. The Cleft Palate-Craniofacial Journal. 2018

[17] Bajaj A, Rao KS, Sharma SM, Shetty V. Modified presurgical nasoalveolar molding in the infants with complete unilateral cleft lip and palate: A stepwise approach. Journal of Oral and Maxillofacial Surgery. 2011;**10**(3):275-280

[18] Priyanka Niranjane P, Kamble RH, Pallavi Diagavane S, Sunita Shrivastav S, Puneet Batra SD, Vasudevan PP. Current status of presurgical infant orthopaedic treatment for cleft lip and palate patients: A critical review. Indian Journal of Plastic Surgery. 2014;**47**(3):293-302

[19] Suri S, Thompson B. A modified muscle-activated maxillary orthopaedic appliance for presurgical nasoalveolar moulding in infants with unilateral cleft lip and palate. Cleft Palate-Craniofacial Journal. 2004;**41**(3):225-229

[20] Rossell-Perry P. The surgical nasoalveolar moulding: A rational treatment for unilateral cleft lip nose deformity and literature review. PRS Global Open. 2020

[21] Batra P et al. OrthoAligner NAM: A case series of Pre-surgical infant orthopedics (PSIO) using clear Aligners. The Cleft Palate-Craniofacial Journal. 2020;**57**(5):646-655

[22] Al Khateeb KA, Fotouh MA, Abdelsayed F, Fahim F. Short-term efficacy of presurgical vacuum formed nasoalveolar molding aligners on nose, lip, and maxillary arch morphology in infants with unilateral cleft lip and palate: A prospective clinical trial. The Cleft-Palate Craniofacial Journal. 2021;**58**(7):815-823

[23] Subramanian CS, Prasad NKKK, Chitharanjan AB, Liou EJW. A modified presurgical orthopedic (nasoalveolar molding) device in the treatment of unilateral cleft lip and palate. European Journal of Dentistry. 2016;**10**(3):435-438

Chapter 2

Perspective Chapter: Role of Genetics, Stem Cells in Reconstructive Surgery—Their Perspectives in Craniofacial Diseases and Syndromes

Surya Sudhakar V. Goparaju

Abstract

Genetic screening, counseling, and mapping play a vital role in identification of mutant genes/chromosomes, thereby preventing the progression of the disease in craniofacial anamolies, head and neck cancer in susceptible patients. Stem cells have a wide application in treating autoimmune diseases and systemic diseases, craniofacial anomalies, head and neck cancers, esthetic and reconstructive surgery, etc. At large, surgery has been the mainstay of treatment in both disease varieties. Targeted therapies with genetic engineering and stem cell transplantation go hand in hand for improving the prognosis of these diseases to a phenomenal extent. The identification of the disease at the level of chromosomal mutation stem cell therapy in conjunction with surgery is a suitable option to obtain satisfactory results in both the disease entities. This methodical combination aids in correction of the relapse and recurrence in craniofacial anomalies as well as head and neck cancers. This chapter projects and encourages insight into the perspective approach and the importance of combining whole genome sequencing and mapping along with stem cell therapy along with the conventional treatment modalities in treatment of craniofacial deformities, head and neck neoplasms with the right timing and proper case selection to appreciate better results.

Keywords: craniofacial anomalies, head and neck cancer, gene mutations and sequencing, stem cell therapy, craniofacial diseases and syndromes

1. Introduction

Craniofacial malformations occur due to the result of an infant's skull or facial bones fusing together very early or in an abnormal way. When the cranial bones fuse together too early, the brain gets conducive in the cranial vault and cannot expand properly due to inadequate space, which causes infant to develop craniofacial deformities and neurological problems. Craniofacial defects like cleft lip and palate, craniosynostosis/syndromes may occur because of congenital anamoly, injury or tumor.

Genetic screening and counseling imparts an immense role in the identification of the causative gene that is responsible for the mutations in craniofacial anomalies through the gene mapping and whole genomic sequencing methods which also helps in controlling the run over of the craniofacial anomalies in future generation among the affected family members. Further step ahead, genetic engineering helps to identify and correct the genetic mutations so as to plan the treatment for the affected patient on a long term basis, to give a better quality of life.

Surgery remains the treatment of choice in correction of craniofacial deformities as well as in reconstruction of craniofacial defects. Genetics and tissue engineering through stem cells have contributed in identification of gene mutations in craniofacial anomalies/syndromes and in their treatment through autologous bone grafting combined with application of stem cells engineered through in vitro and in vivo cell lineage cultures for the reconstruction of craniofacial skeleton.

2. Genetic screening and gene therapy in patients with craniofacial malformations

Genetic screening by a clinical geneticist or genetic counselor plays a pivotal role in determining the patients with isolated craniofacial anomalies and syndromes. The identification of specific syndrome is important for the overall care of the patient as it identifies the risks of other medical problems that will have to be taken into account for the overall well being of the infant as well as in the management of the craniofacial malformation/syndrome. This helps the parents and family members to understand the cause and recurrence risk with future child births. Various methods of genetic testing such as karyotype, fluorescence in situ hybridization, chromosomal microarrays and next generation sequencing can be utilized in doing the genetic screening and mapping.

Karyotype analysis finds the chromosome number and searches for deletions and duplications. The flouroscent in situ hybridisation locates specific minor deletions in genome. The chromosomal microarrays/comparative ggenomic hybridisation focusses on complete genetics at finer detail as compared with other two. Advanced technologies are based on next generation sequencing that throws lighton individual base pairs of DNA encoding proteins [1]. This contains either doing a panel of genes of a specific disorder or whole genome sequencing which is available with genetic testing companies and laboratories that offer panels of genes for specific disorders as well as whole genomic sequencing.

The clinical features of the craniofacial anomalies are peculiar as they can occur as isolated, non syndromic or as a part of Mendelian syndromes. The medical geneticist and genetic counselor determine the type of cases that which are syndromic or isolated. Studies have shown linkage of non-syndromic cleft at region of 9q21, which after subsequent fine mapping revealed the significance of forkhead box protein E1 (FOXE1). It is genetically expressed at the point of fusion between maxillary and nasal process during palate formation whose mutations resulted in cleft palate, in mice studies. The other genes are interferon regulatory factor 6(IRF 6), transforming growth factor –alfa (TGFA). GWASs have confirmed the significance of IRF6 and FOXE1, 8Q24, 10Q25 AND 17Q22 in non- syndromic cleft palate cases.

The syndromes associated with cleft lip and palate include chromosomal abnormalities like trisomy 21, 18, 13, microdeletion syndromes (22q11 deletion syndrome), autosomal dominant disorder like VanderWoude syndrome and single gene disorders. The syndromes of cleft lip alone without cleft palate result from single gene defect which account for 75% and are associated with Mendelian disorders. The cleft lip with palate and cleft palate alone are embyologically separate entity with cleft lip and palate associated with syndromes are 50% and cleft lip alone are up to 75%. The cleft palate phenotype have been identified with chromosomes like Xq21 with TBX22 gene, TBX1gene (Di George/velocardiofacial syndromes). The SATB2 gene was identified as the cause of isolated cleft palate through its role in transcriptional regulation and disruption.

On the other side of the coin, the commonest craniosynostosis syndromes are due to mutation in fibroblast growth factor receptor 2 gene (FGFR2) which alters the protein to prolong signaling such that immature embryonic cell become bone embedded cells which can promote the premature fusion of bones in the skull, hands and feet. The eight known FGFR related craniosynostosis include Crouzon syndrome (with and without acanthosis nigricans), Apert syndrome, Pfeiffer syndrome, Jakson –Weiss syndrome, Beare-Stevenson syndrome, Muenke syndrome etc. Meunke syndrome is caused by gene mutation in FGFR3 gene.

Microtia is associated with gene mutations in syndromes such as Treacher Collin's syndrome (TCOF1, POLR 1C, POLR 1D gene), Nager syndrome (SF3B4, PRX1, PRX2 gene).

The causative gene of these craniofacial disorders/syndromes can be identified by DNA sequencing. The craniofacial malformations that are isolated, as well as that which are associated with genetic syndromes help the subject to be aware of the possible diseases and complications associated with other body systems. Majority of the craniosynostosis and syndromes can be diagnosed based on clinical findings, however, identification of genetic mutations is beneficial to the patients, family members and their next generations [2, 3].

2.1 Gene therapy in craniofacial deformities and regeneration

Conceptually, gene therapy involves insertion of new genetic material into cell to manipulate the endogenous proteins inside the cell. The methods of gene transfer are using DNA either in solution, conjugated to a biomaterial (polymers) or by viruses. In both of these, genes are transferred with in a plasmid that contains the genetic information necessary for the cell to begin making the protein product of that gene once the plasmid enters the nucleus. Viral transduction is the most effective method for gene transfer. The three main classes of viruses used for gene therapy are retroviruses, adeniviruses and adeno associated viruses. Even though the viral transduction is by far thee most effective method for gene transfer, it holds the insidious risk of insertional oncogenesis, toxic immune response, viral replication and dissemination.

Retroviruses are ideal for long term gene therapy, where in, the current human genome contains up to 5–8 of endogenous retroviral sequences that have been acquired over an evolutionary period. Adenoviruses are more suited for short term gene delivery and are used for tissue engineering that require a protein production over several weeks as they are non toxic and self limiting.

Gene therapy has been used to reprogram the fate of cells to generate induced pluripotent stem cells which change to a state of pluripotency and can differentiate to multiple different cell types. Through the insertion of specific genes involved in pluripotency of embryonic stem cells, somatic cells can be reprogrammed into cells that have self renewal and differentiation capabilities and hence are named induced pluripotent stem cells. These cells can regenerate cells from all three germ layers and can be made patient specific that overcomes the ethical issues unlike embryonic stem cells.

Adult stem cells are an excellent choice for reprogramming them into iPS stem cells due to their relative ease of isolation from different tissues, craniofacial region especially such as gingival fibroblasts, dental pulp stem cells. These cells have been successfully reprogrammed into iPS cells since these are ideal donors from the aspect of obtaining their precursor tissue from donor sites such as mandible and third molar teeth [4]. The craniofacially derived stem cells possess epigenetic memory can enhance their differentiating capability towards their tissue of origin and enhance their use for craniofacial reconstruction.

Gene therapy is used to repair and regenerate the complex tissues in craniofacial region as well as in treatment of tumor itself with genetic transfer which has made a significant progress in the last decade. This includes approval of H101 oncolytic adenovirus for treatment of head and neck cancer. Oncolytic viruses work by specifically targetting and replicating in tumor cells to result in cell death and dicrease in overall tumor size. In addition, Onco VEXR, works to regulate the immune response to the tumor by induction of antigen specific T cell responses. Genetic treatments of the tumor itself may limit the subsequent amount of reconstruction required.

In correction of craniofacial deformities, gene therapy can transform cells at the site of injury into protein synthesizing portals towards correcting them [3]. Reterovirus can be delivered directly to the desired site in which host tissue is transduced ex vivo and implanted at the site requiring tissue regeneration. Retrovirus regenerated femoral defects in rats with adenovirus transduced adipose tissue. Like plasmid DNA, viruses can be delivered on biocompatible scaffolds to generate desired protein production and tissue growth through spatial coordination of cells.

Till to date all strategies for whole tooth bioengineering have relied on the use of stem cells derived from dental pulp, periodontal ligament and/or developing tooth germ with very little emphasis on gene delivery. Further studies using recombinant adeno associated virus (AAV) is needed for bone repair due to qualities ofsuperior safety, tissue engineering and in vivo transduction. In vivo AAV mediated expression of constituently active activin receptor like kinase-2 and BMP-7 has enhanced the healing of bone defects in rodent models [5].

3. Application of stem cells in reconstruction of maxillofacial region and treatment of head and neck pathology

Stem cells have a wide application including treating variety of diseases and reconstruction of maxillofacial region, head and neck. Stem cells can be broadly classified into embryonic and adult somatic mesenchymal types. Adult stem cells are categorized into bone marrow, adipose tissue and dental sub varieties. Embryonic stem cells are categorized into somatic and pleuripotent stem cells. Both embryonic and adult stem cells can be further classified into undifferentiated, early differentiated and differentiated stem cells. The early differentiated stem cells from both the above types can be used along with the scaffold in the reconstruction of the surgical defect of maxillofacial region.

Bone marrow and adipose derived stem cells have been used along with autogenous bone grafts as scaffold in jaw reconstruction. Stem cells have been found effective in treatment of oral mucosal lesions, malignancies of the craniofacial region, along with auto immune and systemic diseases as well.

Various clinical trials are in vogue presently regarding the effect of stem cells as a treatment modality. This presentation attempted to focus insight into the application of stem cell therapy in treatment of diseases as well as reconstruction of the maxillofacial region.

Stem cells are building blocks of all organs, tissues, blood and immune system that serve as an internal repair and regeneration. Found in blood, bone marrow, muscle, adipose tissue, skin, heart, liver, placenta, amniotic fluid, membrane and sac. They lie dormant until needed to regenerate the diseased tissue. Adult humans have blood creating stem cells in bone marrow ranging between 50,000 to 2,00,000. They are activated to proliferate and differentiate into required type, upon their loss, thus maintain tissue homeostasis. Various types of stem cells are embryonic, adult, mesenchymal, tissue specific, Induced pluripotent stem cells. The adult stem cell types are hematopoetic, mesenchymal, neural, epithelial, adipose.

4. Cancer stem cells

Cancer stem cells arise from normal somatic stem cells. In the process of normal differentiation, a cell differentiates to form two cells, differentiated and primitive. A terminally differentiated cell is formed from precursor progenitor cell and finally undergoes apoptosis. CSC may originate from a normal stem cell, a normal progenitor cell or a normal differentiated cell by genetic mutation which will activate self renewal genes. During the normal differentiation process of the stem cell, instead of apoptosis, mutations occur in stem cell, progenitor cell and differentiated cell, by which they transform into respective mutated cells, there by resulting in formation of a cancer stem cell. The tumor tissue microenvironment is composed of a variety of cells, including tumor cells, cancer stem cells along with blood vessels. The cancer stem cells are rare cells found primarily in the invasive edge of tumors close to blood vessels [6].

Human cancer tissues are heterogeneous in nature and become differentiated during expansion of cancer stem cells (CSCs). CSCs initiate tumorigenesis, and are involved in tumor recurrence and metastasis. Furthermore, data show that CSCs are highly resistant to anticancer drugs. Human cancer tissues are heterogeneous in nature and become differentiated during expansion of cancer stem cells CSCs). CSCs initiate tumorigenesis, and are involved in tumor recurrence and metastasis. Furthermore, data show that CSCs are highly resistant to anticancer drugs [6].

4.1 Therapeutic targeting strategies for CSCs

Stem cells here play a dual role-in carcinogenesis and in the development of possible new cancer treatment options in future. For past so many years stem cells have been used in the replenishment of blood and immune system damage during treatment of cancer by chemotherapy or radiotherapy. Other than their use in the immuno-reconstitution, the stem cells have been reported to contribute in the tissue regeneration as they have extraordinary capacity to regenerate and differentiate. The MSCs have been used in the cell-based bone reconstruction following chemotherapy and surgery in malignancies like osteosarcoma and Ewing sarcoma [7].

Another important aspect of their use in cancer therapy is the use as delivery vehicle. Systematic delivery of drug or gene therapy has promising future but is currently limited by various factors such as immune detection, nonspecific accumulation in normal tissues and poor permeation. Stem cells can be cell based carriers that target the desired site [7, 8]. Stem cells are also used as delivery vehicles based on the hypothesis that the tumor cells send factors such as Vascular endothelial growth factor, to recruit mesenchymal stem cells from the supporting stroma of the tumor.

New techniques of targeting specific cell membrane growth factor receptors or downstream signaling pathway mutations are currently under investigation, especially in patients with metastatic tumors. One of the most promising strategies for cancer treatment is inhibiting the key self-renewal signaling pathways (e.g. Wnt, SHH, Notch signaling pathways) that are aberrantly active in CSCs, introducing novel therapeutic approaches for HNSCC. These new therapeutic techniques have a significant reduction in the CSCs, reducing its tumorigenicity, apoptotic resistance, and enhanced the sensitivity to Cancer therapy. The markers used to isolate, identify and enrich CSCs such as CD44-HYALURONIC ACID RECEPTOR, CD 24- HEAT STABLE ANTIGEN (for solid tumors), CD133, CD166, Ep CAM etc. are also ideal targets for cancer therapy.

Targeting ATP binding casette transport drugs plus other chemotherapeutic drugs, also offers a very powerful and selective stratcgy to eliminate CSCs. Recent therapeutic strategies exploited the interdependence of CSCs and vascular endothelial cells (perivascular niche) in head and neck cancer to decrease the rate of tumor recurrence and distant metastasis.

Compounds targeting the intrinsic and extrinsic apoptosis pathways are bicyclic cyclohexenones capable for inhibiting NF-jB signaling by inhibiting NF-jB-induced interleukin-8 (IL-8) expression, thus exerting anti-proliferative activity against lung adenocarcinoma epithelial cell line, T cell lymphoblast-like cell line, and prostate carcinoma cell line.

Nuclear factor kappa-light-chain enhancer of activated B cells (NF-jB) is a transcription factor that inhibits apoptosis by elevating the expression of survival factor. Another interesting way to manage tumor progression is inducing the terminal differentiation of CSCs to lose their self renewal property, by the means of either retinoic acids or drugs targeting tumor epigenetic changes.

4.2 Procurement and delivery of stem cells

Stem cells can be derived from the following sources like embryonic stem cells sources and adult stem cells sources. The tissue samples containing stem cells are placed under specific conditions in laboratories/stem cell banks. The extraction of these stem cells is possible due to unique receptors like Oct 4, TRA-1-60 Nanog, SSEA4, TRA-1-60 and TRA-1-81 (stem cell markers) present on the stem cell surface [7]. Tissue samples containing stem cells are placed in a sealed vial containing an appropriate media, which nourishes it during transport. The extracted stem cells are grown on a suitable scaffold medium made of biomaterials (biodegradable or non biodegradable) such as poly lactic acid, polyglycolic acid (PGA), polyethylene terepthalate, polypropylene fumarate, hydroxyapatite/tricalcium phosphate, fibrin, alginates, and collagen polytetrafluoro ethylene, fibrin sealent and certain growth factors that act as matrix during regeneration of the tissue. Stem cells are loaded in an suitable carrier called "scaffold" for transfer to desired site to close the defects or replace the organ. Scaffold can be of different shapes, pattern and biomaterials.

The sample should reach the processing storage facility before 40 hours. In the laboratory the samples were trypsinized and passaged to yield colonies of stem cells. The required cell type can be manipulated by utilizing right inductive signals and appropriate growth factors to the stem cells. Cultured stem cells should be passed through stem cell markers before it is administered to patients to know the lineage of the cell. Endotoxin test should be subjected compulsorily to the cultured stem cells to rule out any microbial contamination [9].

4.3 Mechanism of action of stem cells in defects and diseases of craniofacial region

The key role of stem cell therapy in oral mucosal lesions is primarily aimed at neoangiogenesis, tissue regeneration, increased cellularity, modulation of collagen gene expression and immunomodulation, thus making it a versatile promising treatment modality.

Stem cells are divided into embryonic and adult types. Among these the embryonic stem cells are derived by invitro fertilization, elective abortion, somatic cell nuclear transfer and cloning. The adult stem cells can be obtained from three sources such as [2] bone marrow (subdivided into hematopoetic and mesenchymal), [3] oro facial region (decidous teeth, tooth follicle, buccal mucosa, alveolar bone, periodontal ligament, dental pulp, periosteum) [4] other body tissues (skin, adipose tissue).

At present the stem cell research is focused on treatment of oral mucosal lesions such as oral mucositis, oral ulcers, pemphigus vulgaris, oral lichen planus, submucous fibrosis, oral carcinomas etc. In oral submucous fibrosis it is believed to act in removal of pathologically altered collagen and stimulation of healthy collagen through collagen gene expression and immunomodulation (b) Promoting neoangiogenesis. (c) promoting antioxidant action [7].

5. Overall potential uses of stem cells

1. Serve as repair system for the body-The pluripotent nature allows to divide into more stem cells that can be used to regenerate or repair diseased tissue and organs. Eg: mesenchymal stromal cells accelerate wound healing, by modulating immune response and promoting angiogenesis by releasing chemo cytokines and growth factors.

2. Reconstructive surgery- tissue defects, malformations, esthetics procedures.

    - For treatment of bony and soft tissue defects due to trauma, burns, non healing wounds complicated by ischemia due to diabetes.-Scar revision, skin rejuvination, hair transplantation, breast augmentation.

    - Can reduce surgical risk in elderly patients w.r.t donor site morbidity. -Increase the survival of fat graft by cell assisted lipo-transfer.-Prevent allotransplant rejection by establishing lifelong tolerance- in composite tissue allo transplantation cases in residual defects of trauma, congenital anamolies, tumor ablation etc., thus avoiding the use of immuno suppressive agents.

3. Diseases – To know how diseases occur or why certain cells develop into cancer cells.

Eg: Spinal cord injuries, osteopetrosis, Diabetes type I, Parkinson's, Alzeimer's, Heart and brain stroke, liver and kidney diseases, cancer and osteoarthritis, acute leukemia, CML, CLL, aplastic anemia, refractory anemia, congenital thrombocytopenia, Myelodysplastic syndrome, familial lympho histiocytosis etc. and to elicit causes of genetic defects in cells.

4. Induced pleuripotent stem cells: To grow new cells in a laboratory to replace damaged organs or tissues and body systems by genetic reprogramming (SKIN, BLOOD ETC).

5. Drugs: To test and deliver new drugs for effectiveness to the target area.

5.1 General principles

Autologous stem cell/bone marrow transplantation is healthy. Donor must be at least 18 years and above to give legal informed consent. Transplanted patients are required to live in isolation for 100 days while the new immune system establishes. Regenerative power of stem cells declines with age which can be modualted by food and life style habits. The number of stem cells needed varies with the treatment choice or the number of doses requested. The ideal number is 5–10 million/kg of receipient's weight per transplant dose. The minimum no. is 1–2 million stem cells/kg per transplant dose [10]. The donor's stem cells for an allogenic transplant are given to a chemotherapy/radiotherapy patient. These patients tend to have graft vs. cancer cell effect during allo- transplant. Graft failure happens when immune system rejects donor's stem cells.

If more donor stem cells are available, second transplant or with an infusion of residual lymphocytes from the donor may be done. Donors with kidney diseases such as chronic glomerulo nephritis or polycystic kidney disease, nephrectomy patients and are over 40 years old would not able to donate stem cells.

When stem cells/bone marrow are taken from donor, they must have a similar genetic make up. Usually siblings, or a parent or unrelated person should have same genetic component. The match ratio is 1 in 4(match related donor transplant). Others are unlikely to match. Stem cells from the cord blood can be used for the new born, their siblings and other relatives. Patients with genetic disorders like cystic fibrosis need cells from sibling. There is 1 in 4(25%) chance that any of sibling will have inherited the same two sets of HLA genes as the patient. For a parent to be matched, with the patient, both parents must, by chance have some HLA genes in common with each other. The blood or the cheek swab (saliva) is tested for HLA TYPE for potential donor.

Chronic Graft versus host disease (GVHD) which includes dark skin rash, dry or thickened skin, loss of appetite etc. develops after 100 days of transplant usually, but rarely before 3 months after transplant. Up to 80% success results and more than 5 plus year survival rate has been identified owing it to the compatibility of immune system. The published data shows 23 years of cryopreservation of cord stem cells with more storage life for decades. The damage or failure of stem cells is attributed to DNA damage including telomere shortening, DNA replication and failure of repair.

In treating craniofacial deformities, craniofacial fractures or neoplastic lesions, traditional craniomaxillofacial reconstructive surgery techniques along with application of tissue enigineering and regenerative medicine provide long term adequate results avoiding the sequelae of tissue detrimentation. Studies have also shown that regeneration of bone in critical sized defects with periosteum preservation from a self assembling peptide nanofiber hydrogel with iPSCs. The results showed a marked increase in bone volume after 2–4 weeks with a nanofiber hydrogel scaffold with presence of medullary cavities and capillaries. This study suggests that auto-transplantation of osteoprogenitor cells derived from iPSCs combined with a suitable scaffold would be a good therapy for calvarial bone regeneration [11, 12].

Mesenchymal stem cells have the capacity of modulating the immune response and promote tissue regeneration. They can be harvested from many tissues such as skin, pancreas, heart, brain, lung, kidney, cartilage, tendon and teeth, with bone marrow and adipose tissue being the most common sources. The combination of recombinant human bone morphogenic protein-2&7 with mesenchymal stem cells in correction of cleft alveolus and their long term results is yet to be established [13, 14].

Bone marrow stem cells are considered as gold standard for bone regeneration. These stem cells have potential for osteogenic and chondrogenic differentiation. Bone marrow stem cells are obtained by bone marrow aspiration under local/general anesthesia at posterior superior iliac spine, sternum or by in-vitro cultivated bone marrow stem cells. It has been noted that the in-vitro cell population is less potent than the bone marrow aspirate. It is composed of both mesenchymal and hematopoetic stemcells. The disadvantages of bone marrow stem cells is that, there is an increased risk of surgical infection, donor site pain due to invasive technique, volume deficiency in larger defects which need combination of in-vitro culture cell population which is expensive. Conversely, adipose derived stem cells are more readily available as source and can be rapidly expanded [10].

Several in-vivo studies on bone defect regeneration after cyst enucleation, alveolar cleft sugeries, maxillary sinus floor elevation and augmentation using bone marrow stem cells showed favorable results with increased bone formation compared to traditional methods. It was observed that a scaffold free approach to reconstruction with bone marrow stem cell is safe for alveolar cleft repair, but not indicated in large cleft deficiencies. Bone marrow stem cell populations with in vivo activity along with demineralized bone matrix, platelet derived growth factor in tandem with tricalcium phosphate/hydroxyapatite or platelet rich fibrin composites generating bone repair mechanisms [11, 14].

Adipose derived stem cells are a promising alternative to bone marrow stem cells or traditional autogenous bone grafts. Comprising a high cell to volume than other stem cell categories, adipose stem cells are less sensitive to aging, easy to harvest and apply (isolated stromal vascular fraction) enriched with potent growth factors for improved results. Adipose derived stem cells can directly differentiate into osteoblasts and produce chemokines that are useful in facilitating the forming of endogenous stem cells to the site of bone defect. These stem cells can survive in hypoxic environment unlike mesenchymal stem cells by secreting vascular endothelial growth factor, platelet derived growth factor which promote blood vessel formation and enhance hematopoietic cells to allow the exchange of oygen, nutrients, wastes and growth factors necessary for cell survival. ADSC are negatively impacted by donor age in older population.

The stromal vascular fraction is a single source of a diverse population of cells that include multi-potent stem cells, progenitor cells, endothelial cells, stromal cells, pericytes, peri adipocytes, hematopoetic stem cells and macrophages. This holds a promising future direction in cleft palate and craniofacial bone reconstruction and regeneration [15]. In one clinical trial, stromal vascular fraction/adipose derived stem cells used in maxillary sinus floor elevation showed higher bone mass along with blood vessel formation compared to the control group with only adipose derived stem cells usage. ADSC in stromal vascular fraction have shown plasma membrane derived vesicles in the micro environment which establish inter cellular communication due to secretion of angiogenic molecules like FGF2, PDGF, VEGF, MMP-2, MMP-9 and osteogenic molecules like BMP2, RNA and micro RNA that impact the link with neighboring cells and the whole body. Overall, the ADSC have proved to be a multiple benefactor in safety, application and multiple cell transformation which can be collected in larger amounts in one step surgical procedure which decreases rate of infection.

ADSC are obtained through liposuction aspirate or resection of tissue fragments (buccal pad of fat). There are case reports with successful application of in vitro cultivated ADSC in alveolar cleft reconstruction, that wer seeded with demineralized bovine bone mineral and autologous bone. ADSC transferred by vehicular delivery through biphasic bone substitutes such as hydroxyl apatite-tricalcium phosphate scaffolds, poly-L-lactic acid scaffolds and bilaminate fibrin-agarose hydrogels showed significant bone regeneration compared to autologous bone grafting alone [16].

5.2 Tooth derived stem cells

Tooth derived stem cells are an interesting option in repairing bone defects of oral and dental tissues. These cells possess phenotypic characteristics similar to those of BMSCs, and they have the ability to self-renew and differentiate into multiple cell lineages, which are able to form the dentin-pulp structure when transplanted into immuno-compromised animal models. There are five classes of mesenchymal cell populations such as 1) dental pulpal stem cells 2) exfoliated deciduous teeth stem cells 3) periodontal ligament stem cells 4) dental follicle progenitor stem cells 5) stem cells from apical papilla. Of the above 5, stem cells from deciduous teeth (SHEDs) are easily extracted and isolated. They have high levels of immune stimulating and modulating chemokines, broad and multiple differentiation profile and strong proliferative capacity.

Human exfoliated deciduous teeth (SHEDs) are commonly isolated from patients between 5 and 12 years and are rich in post natal stem cells which could be induced into odontoblasts, osteoblasts, myocytes, adipocytes, and neuron-like cells. Dentin and bone could be formed when the cells are transplanted with bioactive materials in vivo. In addition, tooth derived stem cells participate in the repair and regeneration of non-dental tissues; in fact, these cells can differentiate into various types of cells, including neuron, hair follicle, hepatocyte, and cardiomyocyte like cells. Hydrogels may be a good option as a carrier for bone regeneration due to the osteoconductive characteristics of seeded MSCs as well as other advantages, such as injectability.

Dental pulpal stem cells are isolated from third molar extraction sites from teenage young adults. Both dental pulp stem cells and SHEDs are equally potent in cell regeneration and cultures with high concentration of secretomes (soluble paracrine signaling molecules) which allow for their immunomodulatory, angiogenic and neurogenic activities in vivo. SHEDs have been shown to form calvarial bone in critical size defect experiment as compared to other odontogenic tissue derived cell lines in an FGF-2 primed collagenous hydrogel deprived of oxygen, exhibiting markedly increased intramembranous ossification. Human derived dental pulp stem cells with collagen scaffold have the capacity of mature bone formation in calvarial defects with no graft rejection [17–20].

In vivo implantation of the porous composite scaffolds within a critically sized calvarial defect in a rat showed near complete osseous closure of the defect over 6 weeks. An in vitro amplification for harvested MSCs is almost a necessity due to the relatively low numbers of harvested cells (1 MSC/10 4–10 6 stromal cells).

Bone marrow stromal stem cells have been studied in repair of auricular cartilage and craniofacial defects, when embedded in collagen scaffold [21]. Human adipose derived stem cells (h- ADSC) without any medium were able to correct skeletal defects which clearly showed a bone turn over within 2 weeks and a stimulation of the host's reparative process. It was also noted that the bone morphogenic protein (BMP) modulated the h- ADSC through signaling during bone repair [22, 23].

Cranial suture stem cells (SuSC) isolated from calvarial sutures expressed Axin2, a marker to identify slow-cycling stem cells, which showed the ability of skeletal and cartilage repair. Direct engraftment of sutural stem cells (SuSC) to bone defect provided the benefits for cartilage repair through alteration of BMP signaling, leading the role of these cells in intramemebranous bone formation [24].

Several studies have been conducted in rabbit models for mandibular reconstruction with precise defects by integrating scaffolds such as polyether-ether-ketone (PEEK), fibrin glue, with ADSCs and MSCs transcripted with RUNX2 factor showed satisfactory promising results in terms of increase in new bone thickness, volume, compressive resistance, bone mineral density and content with good masticatory load strength [16, 23, 25].

Preliminary clinical studies have shown successful reconstruction with the combination of autologous bone grafts and human bone derived mesenchymal stem cells (BMSC) followed by distraction osteogenesis, dental implants and prosthodontic restoration. A clinical trial conducted by Gjerde et al. on 11 patients with posterior alveolar ridge resorption, evaluated mandibular regeneration using BMSCs without any additional factors like growth factors or stimulants or scaffolds. The result of this study showed successful ridge augmentation [26].

More clinical studies and trials are anticipated in mandibular and craniofacial reconstruction with larger defects using stem cells which could minimize the morbidity due to autologous bone grafting as well as provide long term results and enhance better living of patient.

6. Role of mesenchymal stem cells in craniofacial deformities/head and neck diseases

Majority of the craniomaxillofacial/head and neck anatomic region are formed from mesenchymal cells. Mesenchymal stem cells derived from dental and nondental sources have been effectively used for regeneration in maxillofacial region like regeneration of periodontium, salivary gland, repair of cleft lip and palate and craniofacial regeneration. These cells promote tissue regeneration and wound healing through synergistic downregulation of proinflammatory cytokines and increased production of soluble factors with antioxidant, anti apoptotic and proangiogenic properties.
In oral wounds, they exhibit increased re-epithelialization, cellularity, intracellular matrix formation and neoangiogenesis, thereby accelerate wound healing. Hence mesenchymal stem cell therapy is a promising modality in healing soft tissue and hard tissue wounds of craniofacial region [7, 27].

Adipose cells with appropriate shaped scaffold can be used for reconstruct stem cells isolated from dental pulp has a potential to differentiate into osteoblasts and are a good source for bone formation. Stem cells from oral and maxillofacial region sub sites can be combined with bone marrow stem cells to correct larger defects. Oromaxillofacial bone tissue repair with stem cells was done using collagen sponge scaffold and dental pulp stem cells [9].

Scaffold free tissue constructs to close the critical size bone defects can be used in the form of microspheres. It was found that, osteogenically differentiated microspheres with outgrowing cells can be used to fill up bone defects. This new procedure has added advantage of permitting the transplantation of more cells and better integrity compared with cell suspensions or gels ion of soft tissues. Autologous fibrin glue that holds the cells in place was prepared by cryoprecipitation. This successful technique has given new rays of hope that ADSCs can be used for difficult reconstructive procedures of craniofacial defects [9].

Mesenchymal stem cells (MSCs) are multipotent stromal cells that are present in most adult connective tissues. MSCs have been widely used in stem cell transplantation, tissue engineering, gene therapy, and immunotherapy. These cells express CD105, CD73, andCD90, and are not able to express CD45, CD34, CD14, orCD11b, CD79α or CD19 antigens. In addition, they are able to differentiate into at least 3 cell lineages (immune modulatory, angiogenesis and antiapoptosis effects) in vitro, including chondroblasts, osteoblasts, and adipocytes.

MSC reduce IL-6, tumor necrosis factor-α (TNF-α), and IL-1β levels, 3 days after fracture. This process leads to a better regeneration by limiting tissue injury and inhibiting the progression of fibrosis. The production of inflammatory cytokines, including TNF –alfa, IL-6, IL-12p 70, and IFN-gamma, by macrophages is significantly suppressed by MSCs, while the production of anti-inflammatory cytokines like IL-10 and IL-12p40 is increased. Possibly PGE2 is the key mediator for this process [1]. The anti-apoptotic effect of MSCs could also accelerate the process of bone healing. It has been suggested that faster bone healing with MSC transplantation may be especially correlated with lower levels of TNF-α expression in the callus. This may favor bone formation since it has been reported that TNF-α can have pro-apoptotic effects on osteoblasts [1, 7].

6.1 Tissue engineering approaches with stem cells

In larger bone defects the local injection of stem cells is ineffective. Controlled delivery of MSCs to the desired site is achieved by three ways [2]. Delivery of cells within injectable or prefabricated scaffolds, [3] co-delivery of cells with osteoinductive growth factors or co-culture with other cell types, and [4] Delivery of cells within a 3D dynamic environment. A refabricated bone requires 3 elements, scaffolds or carriers (a 3D support), endothelial growth factors9stimulation of neovascularisation and provision of blood supply) and, MSCs and other growth promotion factors (stimulus for osteoinduction and recruitment of endogenous MSCs). An ideal scaffold/carrier should have four charecteristics, including osteogenesis, osteoincorporation, osteoinduction and osteoconduction [10].

Co-delivery of mesenchymal stem cells with prefabricated 3 dimensional scaffolds along with growth factors that possess properties of osteogenesis, osteoincorporation, osteoinduction, osteoconduction yields better results.

Future directions: A team of professionals including stem cell biologists, molecular biologists, geneticists, polymer and materials scientists, mechanical engineers and clinicians with knowledge of oral and maxillofacial disorders is needed to develop the field of craniofacial tissue engineering.

DOI: http://dx.doi.org/10.5772/intechopen.109514

Though the stem cells and gene therapy have been used in experimental animal studies, it is a major challenge to accomplish regeneration of tissues and vascularity in larger craniofacial defects, as the cells must be within 100mu.m of an oxygen source to survive. In addition to vascular supply, accurate craniofacial reconstruction demands production of tissue interface to repair structures such as joint, tooth and muscle attachments. Use of gene transfer to engineer a cell in producing protein for tissue repair overcomes limitations of recombinant protein therapy in craniofacial regeneration. Somatic cells can be genetically corrected and re-programmed into iPS stem cells that in turn differentiate into disease free cells. Gene therapy in combination with iPS cell technology has great potential use in treating congenital disorders.

Application of stem cells in craniofacial regeneration and reconstruction should be transmuted from animal models to more number human case studies and clinical trials since substantial evidence is available through animal model studies regarding their results in craniofacial regeneration. Targeted tissue engineering therapy for reconstruction of defects and deformities in various sub-units of cranio-facial skeleton with the following illustrated methodology can yield more promising results in the future.- Calvarial bone regeneration through induced pluripotent stem cells delivered by hydrogel injectable system; Cartilagenous regeneration within nasal complex with cranial suture derived stromal stem cells; Maxillary and palatal bone regeneration by mesenchymal (adipose or bone marrow derived) stem cell delivery; Mandibular defect regeneration by polyether ether ketone (PEEK) scaffold delivery of mesenchymal stem cells. Particularly of more interest is the potency of developing induced pluripotent stem cells into specific cell lineage of requirement by selectively tuning the gene expression through genetic engineering. So far fundamentally, ADSCs and BMSCs have been successful as stem cell lineages in both pre-clinical and human clinical trials, more so are ADSCs in terms of bone regeneration. Stem cells have the dual capacity as cell based carrier for drug delivery as well as gene therapy. Insightful further research is required to understand the role of stem cells in cancer therapies, with the eventual goal of eliminating the residual disease and recurrence.

Summary

Autologous bone grafting has been the gold standard so far in the reconstruction of craniofacial defects and deformities. Future direction must point out towards application of stem cells for reconstruction of craniofacial defects and deformities of larger volume, thus minimizing the donor site morbidity caused by autologous hard and soft tissue grafting.

Author details

Surya Sudhakar V. Goparaju
Department of Oral and Maxillofacial Surgery, Mamata Dental, Medical College and General Hospital, Khammam, Telangana, India

*Address all correspondence to: sudhakargvs@yahoo.com

References

[1] Fitzsimmons REB et al. Mesenchymal stromal/stem cells in regenerative medicine and tissue engineering. Stem Cells International. 2018;**2018**:8031718

[2] Yoon AJ, Pham BN, Dimple KM. Genetic screening in patients with craniofacial malformations. Journal of Pediatric Genetics. 2016;**5**(4):220-223. DOI: 10.1055/s-0036-1592423

[3] Scheller EL et al. Gene therapy: Implications for craniofacial regeneration. The Journal of Craniofacial Surgery. 2012;**23**(1):333-337. DOI: 10.1097/SCS.0b013e318241dc11

[4] Saito A et al. Targeted reversion of induced pluripotent stem cells from patients with human c leidocanial dysplasia improves bone regeneration in rat calvarial bone defects. Tissue Engineering. Part A. 2012;**18**:1479-1489

[5] Marazita ML. The evolution of human genetic studies of cleft lip and cleft palate. Annual Review of Genomics and Human Genetics. 2012;**13**:263-283

[6] Ohnishi Y et al. Molecularly-targeted therapyfor the oralcancer stem cells. Japanese Dental Science Review. 2018;**54**:88-103

[7] Suma GN, Arora MP, Lakhanpal M. Stem cell therapy: A novel treatment approach for oral mucosal lesions. Journal of Pharmacy & Bioallied Sciences. 2015;**7**(1):2-8. DOI: 10.4103/0975-7406.149809

[8] Baniebrahimi G, Mir F, Khanmohammad R. Cancer stem cells and oral cancer: Insights into molecular mechanisms and therapeutic approaches. Cancer Cell International. 2020;**20**:113. DOI: 10.1186/s12935-020-01192-0

[9] Sunil PM, Manikandhan R, Muthu MS, Abraham S. Stem cell therapy in oral and maxillofacial region: An overview. Journal of Oral and Maxillofacial Pathology. 2012;**16**(1):58-62

[10] Wu V et al. Bone tissue regeneration in the oral and maxillofacial region: A review on the application of stem cells and new strategies to improve vascularization. Stem Cells International. 2019;**2019**:6279721

[11] Behnia H et al. Secondary repair of alveolar clefts using human mesenchymal stem cells. Oral Surgery, Oral Medicine, Oral Pathology, Oral Radiology and Endodontology. 2009;**108**:e1-e6

[12] Mohammed EEA et al. Osteogenic differentiation potential of human bone marrow and amniotic fluids-derived mesenchymal stem cells in vitro & in vivo. Open Access Maced. J. Med. Sci. 2019;7:507-515

[13] Gladysz D et al. Stem cell regenerative therapy in alveolar cleft reconstruction. Archives of Oral Biology. 2015;**60**:1517-1532

[14] Fallucco MA et al. Primary reconstruction of alveolar clefts using recombinant human bone morphogenic protein-2: Clinical and radiographic outcomes. The Journal of Craniofacial Surgery. 2009;**20**:1759-1764

[15] Conejero JA, Lee JA, Parrett BM, et al. Repair of palatal bone defects using osteogenically differentiated fat-derived stem cells. Plastic and Reconstructive Surgery. 2006;**117**:857-853

[16] Fang D, Roskies M, et al. Three dimensional printed scaffolds with

multipotent mesenchymal stromal cells for rabbit mandibular reconstruction and engineering. Methods in Molecular Biology. 2017;**1553**:273-291

[17] Novais A et al. Priming dental pulp stem cells from human exfoliated deciduous teeth with fibroblast growth factor-2 enhances mineralization within tissue engineered constructs implanted I craniofacial bone defects. Stem Cells Translational Medicine. 2019;**8**:844-857

[18] Kichenbrand C, Velot E, Menu P, et al. Dental pulp stem cell-derived conditioned medium: An attractive alternative for regenerative therapy. Tissue Engineering. Part B, Reviews. 2019;**25**:78-88

[19] Lei Y, Jeong D, Xiao J, Schaffer DV. Developing defined and scalable 3D culture systems for culturing human pluripotent stem cells at high densities. Cellular and Molecular Bioengineering. 2014;7:172-183

[20] Riccio M, Maraldi T, Pisciotta A, et al. Fibroin scaffold repairs critical size bone defects in vivo supported by human amniotic fluid and dental pulp stem cells. Tissue Engineering. Part A. 2012;**18**:1006-1013

[21] Baptista LS et al. Adult stem cells spheroids to optimize cell colonization in scaffolds for cartilage and bone tissue engineering. International Journal of Molecular Sciences. 2018;**19**:1285

[22] Al-Ahmady HH, Abd Elazeem AF, et al. Combining autologous bone marrow mononuclear cells seeded on collagen sponge with Nano hydroxyapatite and platelet rich fibrin: Reporting a novel strategy for aloveolar cleft bone regeneration. Journal of Cranio-Maxillofacial Surgery. 2018;**46**:1593-1600

[23] Levi B, James AW, Gupta A, et al. Human adipose derived stromal cells heal critical size mouse calvarial defects. PLoS One. 2010;**5**:e11177

[24] Maruyama T, Jeong J, Sheu TJ, Hsu W. Stem cells of the suture mesenchyme in craniofacial bone development, repair and regeneration. Nature Communications. 2016;**7**:10526

[25] Meherbani D, Khodakarm-Tafti A, et al. Comparison of the regenerative effect of adipose- derived stem cells, fibrin glue scaffold and autologous bone graft in experimental mandibular defect in rabbit. Dental Traumatology. 2018;**34**:413-420

[26] Gjerde C, Mustafa K, et al. Cell therapy induced regeneration of severely atrophied mandibular bone in a clinical trial. Stem Cell Research & Therapy. 2018;**9**:213

[27] Oliver JD et al. Stem cell regenerating the craniofacial skeleton: Current state-of- the- art and future directions. Journal of Clinical Medicine. 2020;**9**:3307. DOI: 10.3390/jcm 9103307

Chapter 3

Tissue Induction in Plastic and Maxillo-Facial Surgery

Simone La Padula, Rosita Pensato, Rebecca Sabban, Francesco D'Andrea, Edoardo Coiante, Giovanni Roccaro, Mounia SidAhmed-Mezi, Jean Paul Meningaud and Barbara Hersant

Abstract

Tissue induction is defined as the activation of cell regeneration to restore damaged tissue, which involves stimulating cell signaling and modifying the micro-environment. Tissue inducers therefore have the advantage of acting quickly and durably on treated tissues, alone or in combination with surgical procedures, in order to reduce iatrogeny and potentiate surgical results. The aim of this review was to detail the various current techniques for tissue regeneration in the field of plastic and maxillo-facial surgery. We conducted a systematic search on Pubmed, Google Scholar and Science Direct. Articles in English and French, published after 2012 and focusing on facial tissue induction were searched. Only prospective comparative studies assessing as many cases as possible were analyzed. The following keywords were used: "skin rejuvenation", "skin regeneration", "collagen induction", "skin enhancer", "aging rejuvenation", "oral mucosa rejuvenation", "oral mucosa regeneration", "buccal mucosa rejuvenation", "buccal mucosa regeneration", "oral bone regeneration", "alveolar bone regeneration". Fifty innovative articles published since 2012 dealing with tissue induction techniques with an interest in plastic and maxillo-facial surgery were identified and then selected. The most effective tissue inducers for skin and mucosal regeneration were lasers, radiofrequency, pulsed light, hyaluronic acid and PRP. Tissue induction allows collagen self-production leading to tissue regeneration. Many techniques can be used for tissue induction that represent an additional tool in the therapeutic arsenal available to plastic and maxillofacial surgeons to improve patient management.These inducers can be used alone or in combination to achieve synergistic effects and better clinical outcomes.

Keywords: skin rejuvenation, skin regeneration, oral mucosa regeneration, oral bone regeneration, skin enhancer

1. Introduction

Tissue induction is defined as the activation of collagen self-production allowing quantitative and qualitative tissue regeneration [1–15]. Many techniques are used for tissue induction, especially in the field of skin, mucosa and bone healing and in the field of facial rejuvenation. Tissue inducers may be biological, physical, chemical or mechanical agents. Mechanotransduction is one of these tissue induction processes whose main techniques include needling, osteotensors, massage (LPG), HIFU ultrasound and radiofrequency. They act on dermal fibroblast mechanoreceptors by causing the release of growth factors and therefore an endogenous production of collagen. Tissue induction by photo-biomodulation is mainly based on two techniques, laser therapy and low-level light therapy (LLLT) and acts by modulating collagen production without adverse thermal effect. Cryotherapy is a mode of tissue induction based on the biophysical properties of cold to induce collagen production after short and repeated exposures to a cooling. Tissue induction by bio-induction may be performed by adipose tissue injection or lipofilling, mesenchymal stem cell-enriched and/or platelet-rich plasma (PRP)-enriched adipose tissue injection, filler injection with hyaluronic acid, direct PRP injection and mesotherapy. Resorbable and non-resorbable threads, commonly used as a non-surgical rejuvenation method, especially in the midface region, promote collagen production and can therefore be considered mechanical inducers. The aim of this review was to detail the techniques available for tissue regeneration in the field of plastic and maxillo-facial surgery.

2. Materials and methods

Articles in English or French, published after 2012 and focusing on facial tissue induction were searched on Pubmed Google Scholar and Science Direct. Only prospective comparative studies assessing as many cases as possible were analyzed. The following keywords were used: "skin rejuvenation", "skin regeneration", "collagen induction", "skin enhancer", "aging rejuvenation", "oral mucosa rejuvenation", "oral mucosa regeneration", "buccal mucosa rejuvenation", "buccal mucosa regeneration", "oral bone regeneration", "alveolar bone regeneration". Articles were included if they dealt with one or more cutaneous and mucosal tissue induction techniques for rejuvenation or regeneration on at least five human patients after reading the abstract and the full article. Exclusion criteria: literature reviews, meta-analyses and case studies were excluded, as well as animal experiments and in vitro research. Articles not dealing with tissue induction after complete article reading were also excluded from the study.

3. Results

Case reposts, reviews, animal studies, non-English/French language articles, and off topic papers were excluded (**Figure 1**).

Fifty innovative articles published since 2012 dealing with tissue induction techniques with an interest in plastic and maxillo-facial surgery were identified and then selected [1–10]. Of these articles, 23 dealt with induction techniques for *esthetic* facial rejuvenation and 27 dealt with oral mucosa regeneration techniques. Laser techniques for *esthetic* facial skin rejuvenation were addressed in the greatest number of articles, i.e. 10 articles published since 2012 including six that concluded that the technique was effective. Radiofrequency was addressed in eight articles published since 2012 including six that concluded that the technique was effective on skin rejuvenation. Light therapy was studied in five articles that all showed a significant inducing effect

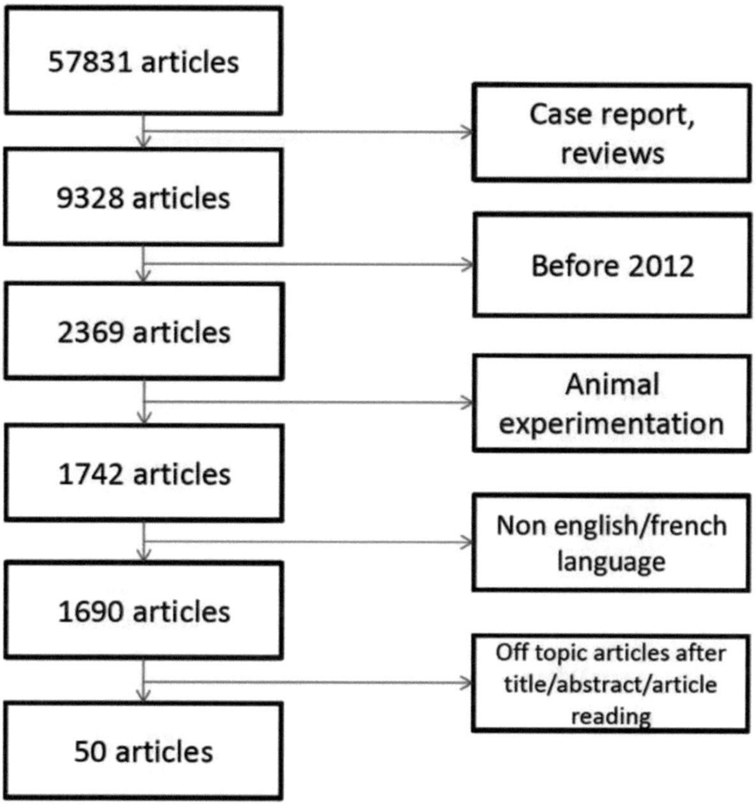

Figure 1.
Flow chart: articles selection.

on tissues. Lipofilling was studied in three articles but only one showed a significant inducing effect on tissues. Finally, mechanostimulation was only studied in one article that concluded to a tissue inducing effect on skin rejuvenation. In the field of facial mucosa and bone healing, the application of PRP or PRP derivatives such as fibrin-rich plasma (FRP) was the most studied technique with 20 articles published since 2012 that all showed an inducing effect on mucosa and bone tissues. The study of the impact of bone stem cell transplantation was more recent with three articles published since 2012 including two that showed positive results. The effect of laser phototherapy on bone regeneration was little studied with only one article published since 2012 but it showed a significant inducing effect on tissues. Similarly, the effect of osteotensors was only studied in one article that showed a non-significant inducing effect on bone tissues. The effect of laser phototherapy on oral mucosa regeneration was studied in one article that concluded to a significant effect on oral mucosa regeneration after surgery.

3.1 Soft tissue induction

Several techniques have been used in the last years to improve the skin aging signs and the soft tissues quality, especially in burn patients [1, 2] The most studied technique is non-ablative Nd:YAG laser. The article by Hong published in 2015 has histologically assessed the efficacy of Nd:YAG laser (1064 nm) on the signs of skin aging such as wrinkles and skin laxity and on the production of dermal collagen in a series of 20 cases [1]. It has shown that after three monthly sessions including three passages on the treated hemiface, with a delivered energy of 20–24 J/cm^3, the number of wrinkles was significantly improved with a 45.1% decrease ($p < 0.001$). The histological assessment corroborated the clinical results with a marked increase in dermal collagen and elastic fibers. Charles-de-Sá et al. [2] have compared the effects of trophic (and non-volumizing) adipose transplantation to those of adipose-derived stem cell transplantation on facial skin rejuvenation. Their protocol was based on the reinjection of autologous fat taken from the abdomen in a hemiface and the reinjection of adipose-derived stem cells, previously isolated and then cultured in the presence of growth factors, in the other hemiface. The final assessment, including a 3-month histological analysis of the reticular dermis arrangement and the number of elastic and collagen fibers, showed an increased density of the collagen and elastin network, the presence of a richer microvascular bed without showing any difference between the two treated areas. Thus, the lipofilling technique appeared to have the same rejuvenating effect as stem cell transplantation without its associated technical complexities. This effect could be explained by the high concentration of mesenchymal stem cells contained in the adipose tissue. Humbert [3] has studied the effect of mechanotransduction on the expression of genes involved in skin regeneration. After a total of 24 sessions of standardized massage on a randomly chosen hemiface in 30 subjects, there was an increase in histological criteria for tissue induction such as the fibroblast migration capacity, showing their activation, an increased synthesis of elastin fibers, endogenous hyaluronic acid and metalloproteases, including MMP9, MMP1 and TIMP1. This study has also shown a 100% patient satisfaction with the anti-aging effect of mechanostimulation with an absence of side effects such as pain. Seo et al. [4] have analyzed the effect of radiofrequency, combined or not with the injection of adipose-derived stem cells, on facial anti-aging rejuvenation. The care protocol included three radiofrequency sessions 1 month apart. The authors have shown an improvement in skin thickness in both groups, which was confirmed by the histological analysis. The latter showed a significant increase in the dermis thickness associated with an increase in collagen fibers and type I pro-collagen after three radiofrequency sessions.

3.2 Bone induction

In his study, Hauser [5] has shown the impact of platelet rich fibrin (PRF) on alveolar bone regeneration. The protocol was based on the addition of autologous PRF in the dental extraction cavity of 23 patients and then a histological analysis of the newly formed alveolar bone 8 weeks after treatment. The microscopic examination showed the creation of a significant bone micro-trabeculation and the maintenance of a bone height significantly higher than in the control group. The results obtained were substantially identical to those obtained with a mucosal coverage flap. This technique could therefore be an alternative to mucosal coverage flaps that are necessary in certain circumstances but could lead to morbidity on the sampling sites. The 2013 study by Kaigler [6] has examined the benefit of bone stem cell transplantation on facial bone defects. Iliac crest bone marrow-derived stem cells were collected, isolated, cultured and reimplanted in areas of mandibular bone defects such as dental extraction cavities. Bone regeneration was measured radiologically and histologically. It showed a better healing with a lesser need for subsequent bone grafting and a significantly greater radiological bone gain in the test group. Histologically, the newly formed bone was denser and more voluminous in the test group. This technique could replace bone transplantation in maxillo-facial surgery in the context of bone defects, a fortiori in case of debilitated backgrounds including after irradiation, while decreasing the morbidity and sequelae of donor sites. In 2015, Odin et al. have studied pre-implant bone tissue induction by mechanotransduction with a protocol of osteotensors in a patient with ectodermal dysplasia [7]. The protocol was based on mechanotherapy sessions for 3–6 weeks before placing dental implants. This technique, through the creation of a transmatricial canal between the periosteum and the endoste with a manual or rotary instrument could activate osteogenesis and angiogenesis through the recruitment of bone stem cells. The 3-year clinical assessment showed a perfect integration of implants and the radiological assessment by Cone-Beam showed a gain in maxillary and mandibular bone height and thickness.

The osteotensor is a flapless mechanotherapy, with creation of a transmatrix channel ranging in size from 200 to 500 μm that sets up communication pathways between the endosteum, the bone marrow, and the periosteum. The resultant bone distraction phenomenon leads to modification of internal bone matrix tensions. This activation causes cell mobilization locally, in the periosteum, endosteum, bone marrow, and along the vascular walls where progenitor cells are recruited. Formation of a blot clot followed by a bony callus reinforces the local architecture. In the sinus regions, where bone is initially type IV, this generally results in transformation into active type II bone. Bleeding under the Schneiderian membrane has a balloon-like effect that elevates the membrane, allowing formation of a callus and a bone gain of 2 to 6 mm.

Romão et al. have studied the effect of laser phototherapy on alveolar bone repair in 20 patients after dental extraction through a radiological and histological assessment [8]. At 40 days, it has been shown both radiologically and histologically that laser phototherapy significantly increased bone thickness and volume after dental extraction and therefore improved bone healing in pre-implant contexts.

4. Discussion

Various tissue induction techniques have been studied and developed in plastic and maxillo-facial surgery. In facial rejuvenation, the most relevant tissue inducers appear to be Nd:YAG laser, trophic lipofilling, mechanostimulation and radiofrequency. Regarding bone induction in maxillo-facial surgery for acquired or congenital defects, the inducers with a proven efficacy are the PRF and the reinjection of bone stem cells. The use of osteotensors should be more carefully studied before being added to the therapeutic arsenal of maxillo-facial surgeons. Many other induction methods are known, but their efficacy has not yet been proved in the plastic and maxillo-facial surgery field [1–15]. Radiofrequency and the plasma (a physical agent) are for example being assessed in non-surgical blepharoplasty. The authors have identified and resumed two main tissue induction mechanisms that act directly and indirectly (**Figures 2** and **3**).

5. Conclusions

Tissue induction allows collagen self-production leading to tissue regeneration. Many techniques can be used for tissue induction that represent an additional tool in the therapeutic arsenal available to plastic and maxillofacial surgeons to improve patient management.

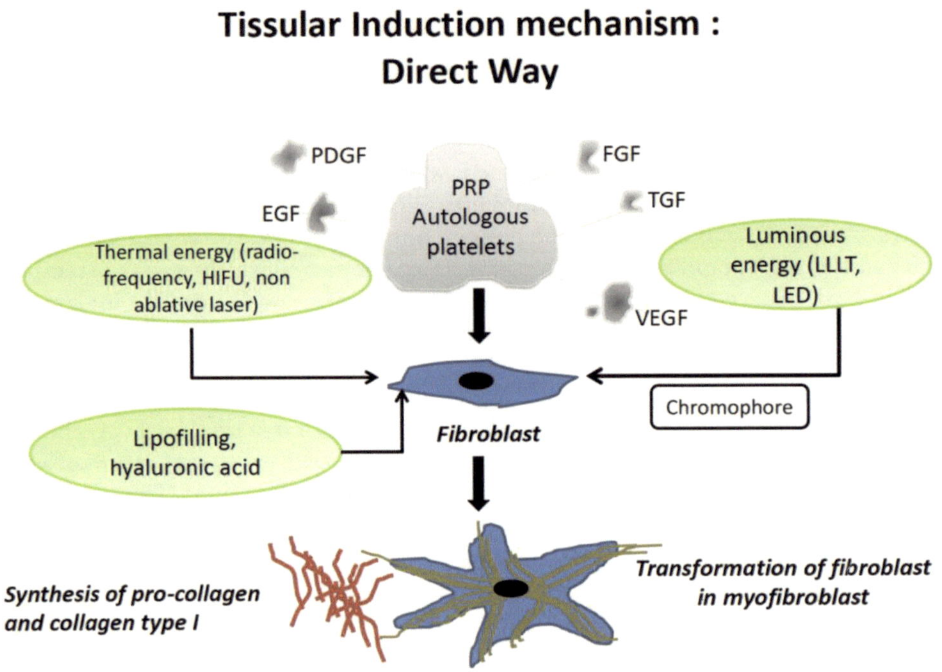

Figure 2.
Activation of fibroblast via PRP after releasing of TGF, EGF, VEGF and FGF thanks to the PDGF. Activation of fibroblast via luminous energy by activation of fibroblastic chromophore and increase synthesis of FGF by macrophages. The peak of efficiency is reached with a wave length including 680 and 840 nm.

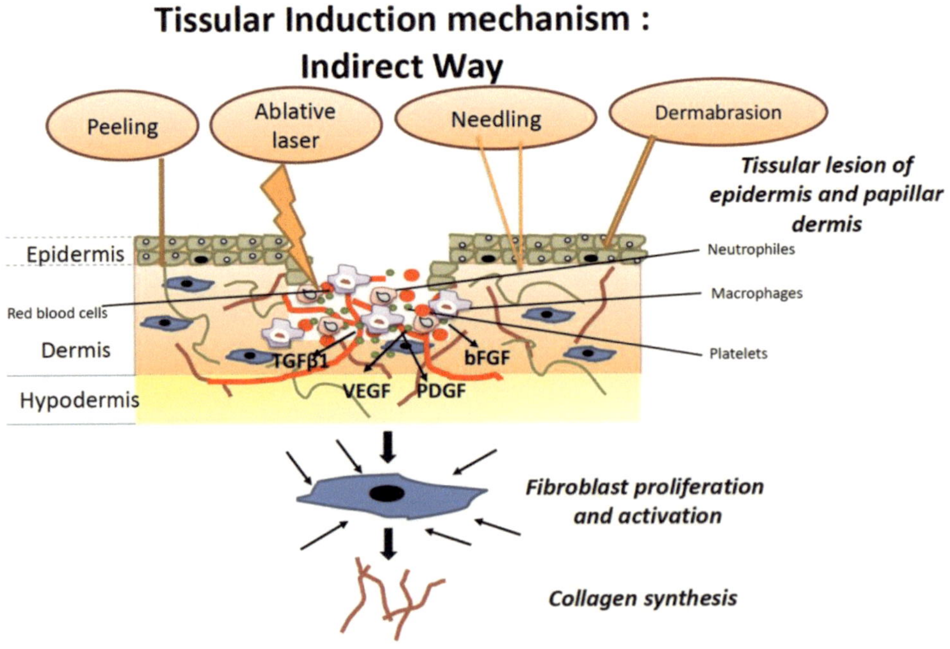

Figure 3.
Tissular lesion of the skin: wound healing process, releasing of growth factors and activation of fibroblasts and collagen synthesis.

Acknowledgements

All the authors have contributed to the writing of this paper.

Funding

This research received no external funding.

Conflicts of interest

The authors declare no conflict of interest.

Data availability statement

Pubmed Google Scholar and Science Direct. No copyright needed.

Author details

Simone La Padula[1,2*], Rosita Pensato[2], Rebecca Sabban[1], Francesco D'Andrea[2], Edoardo Coiante[1], Giovanni Roccaro[1], Mounia SidAhmed-Mezi[1], Jean Paul Meningaud[1] and Barbara Hersant[1]

1 Department of Plastic, Reconstructive and Maxillo facial Surgery, Henri Mondor Hospital, University Paris XII, Créteil, France

2 Department of Plastic and Reconstructive Surgery, Università degli studi di Napoli Federico II, Napoli, Italy

*Address all correspondence to: drsimonelapadula@gmail.com

References

[1] Hong JS, Park SY, Seo KK, Goo BL, Hwang EJ, Park GY, et al. Long pulsed 1064 nm Nd:YAG laser treatment for wrinkle reduction and skin laxity: Evaluation of new parameters. International Journal of Dermatology. 2015;**54**(9):345-350

[2] Charles-de-Sá L, Gontijo-de-Amorim NF, Maeda Takiya C, Borojevic R, Benati D, Bernardi P, et al. Antiaging treatment of the facial skin by fat graft and adipose-derived stem cells. Plastic and Reconstructive Surgery. 2015;**135**(4):999-1009

[3] Humbert P, Fanian F, Lihoreau T, Jeudy A, Elkhyat A, Robin S, et al. Mécano-Stimulation TM of the skin improves sagging score and induces beneficial functional modification of the fibroblasts: Clinical, biological, and histological evaluations. Clinical Interventions in Aging. 2015;**10**:387-403

[4] Seo KY, Kim DH, Lee SE, Yoon MS, Lee HJ. Skin rejuvenation by microneedle fractional radiofrequency and a human stem cell conditioned medium in Asian skin: A randomized controlled investigator blinded split-face study. J Cosmet Laser Ther Off Publ Eur Soc Laser Dermatol. 2013;**15**(1):25-33

[5] Hauser F, Gaydarov N, Badoud I, Vazquez L, Bernard J-P, Ammann P. Clinical and histological evaluation of postextraction platelet-rich fibrin socket filling: a prospective randomized controlled study. Implant Dentistry. 2013;**22**(3):295-303

[6] Kaigler D, Pagni G, Park CH, Braun TM, Holman LA, Yi E, et al. Stem cell therapy for craniofacial bone regeneration: A randomized, controlled feasibility trial. Cell Transplantation. 2013;**22**(5):767-777

[7] Odin G, Petitbois R, Cotten P, Philip P. Distraction osteogenesis using bone matrix osteotensors in ectodermal dysplasia: A case report. Implant Dentistry. 2015;**24**(5):612-619

[8] Romão MM, Marques MM, Cortes AR, Horliana AC, Moreira MS, Lascala CA. Micro-computed tomography and histomorphometric analysis of human alveolar bone repair induced by laser phototherapy: A pilot study. International Journal of Oral and Maxillofacial Surgery. 2015;**44**(12):1521, 8

[9] Hersant B, SidAhmed-Mezi M, Aboud C, Niddam J, Levy S, Mernier T, et al. Synergistic effects of autologous platelet-rich plasma and hyaluronic acid injections on facial skin rejuvenation. Aesthetic Surgery Journal. 2021;**41**(7):NP854-NP865

[10] La Padula S, Hersant B, Pizza C, Chesné C, Jamin A, Ben Mosbah I, et al. Striae distensae: In vitro study and assessment of combined treatment with sodium ascorbate and platelet-rich plasma on fibroblasts. Aesthetic Plastic Surgery. 2021;**45**(3):1282-1293

[11] La Padula S, Hersant B, Noel W, Niddam J, Hermeziu O, Bouhassira J, et al. Use of the retrograde limb of the internal mammary vein to avoid venous congestion in DIEP flap breast reconstruction: Further evidences of a reliable and time sparing procedure. Microsurgery. 2016;**36**(6):447-452

[12] La Padula S, Hersant B, Meningaud JP. Intraoperative use of indocyanine green angiography for selecting the more reliable perforator of the anterolateral thigh flap: A comparison study. Microsurgery. 2018;**38**(7):738-744

[13] Ruiz R, Hersant B, La Padula S, Meningaud JP. Facelifts: Improving the long-term outcomes of lower face and neck rejuvenation surgery: The lower face and neck rejuvenation combined method. Journal of Cranio-Maxillo-Facial Surgery. 2018;**46**(4):697-704

[14] La Padula S, Hersant B, Chatel H, Aguilar P, Bosc R, Roccaro G, et al. One-step facial feminization surgery: The importance of a custom-made preoperative planning and patient satisfaction assessment. Journal of Plastic, Reconstructive & Aesthetic Surgery. 2019;**72**(10):1694-1699

[15] Hersant B, SidAhmed-Mezi M, La Padula S, Niddam J, Bouhassira J, Meningaud JP. Efficacy of autologous platelet-rich plasma glue in weight loss sequelae surgery and breast reduction: A prospective study. Plastic and Reconstructive Surgery. Global Open. 2016. 15;**4**(11):e871

Chapter 4

PRF and Sticky Bone as Regenerative Materials in Oral Surgery

Naida Hadziabdic

Abstract

Platelet-rich fibrin (PRF) as a biological scaffold is attracting clinicians' attention, mainly because it promotes bone and soft tissue healing. As autologous material, PRF has many advantages over other platelet concentrates, such as Platelet-rich plasma (PRP) and Plasma rich in growth factors (PRGF). Among many benefits, simple preparation (centrifugation protocol) stands out because no additional anticoagulant is added to the tubes. This chapter aims to clarify the PRF membranes and sticky bone preparation together with other platelet concentrates. A few clinical cases will show how sticky bone is together with PRF membranes applicative in different oral surgery indications. Clinical and radiological check-ups demonstrated excellent therapeutic outcomes. Sticky bone and PRF membranes have regenerative potential and are advised to use in many oral surgery procedures.

Keywords: platelet concentrates, platelet-rich fibrin, PRF, sticky bone, mineralized plasmatic matrix, concentrated growth factors–enriched bone graft matrix

1. Introduction

Modern times bring many challenges in different life spheres, and medical treatment is not an exception. As dentists, we encounter constant scientific as well as technological developments, and it is with great eagerness that we strive to be active users of these benefits, thereby actively advocating for patients' best care. It is not with ease that a modern man would come to peace with the information that they are not eligible for a particular treatment; in dentistry, for instance, that may be the case when one does not have enough available bone for implants to be placed. This further motivates dentists to replace lost tissues by utilizing regenerative procedures. The principle of regenerative medicine and dentistry is founded on its interdisciplinarity as well as on the application of bioengineering techniques that enable the replacement of any lost tissue. In the field of oral surgery, a branch of dentistry, the most interesting tissue replacement is bone and soft (gingival) tissue replacement [1].

Of great help in regenerative procedures is the application of platelet concentrates that originate from the patient's blood [2]. The role of platelet concentrates in regenerative dentistry is based on the fact that they contain growth factors and scaffolds.

In this chapter, we will be discussing platelet-rich fibrin (PRF) and sticky bone, their preparation techniques, and usage indications. We will hereby also comment on other platelet concentrates.

2. A brief review of platelets and their role in the body

Blood is a liquid tissue that consists of plasma (55%), red blood cells (or erythrocytes 45%), platelets (thrombocytes), and white blood cells (leukocytes) that together account for less than 1%. In the organism, blood acts as a transporting medium, participates in coagulation, and serves as a medium for information transduction (e.g., hormones) [3].

In regenerative processes, the focus is placed on platelets. They originate from megakaryocytes in the blood marrow. Platelets are small, discoid-shaped plate-like cells that have no nucleus and have a lifespan of 8–12 days in a resting state. Apart from their role in hemostasis, they also have a role in inflammatory reactions, wound healing, host defense, and tumor biology [4].

Platelets contain three types of granules (alpha, dense, and lysosomes) that dictate platelets' function. Among the three types of granules, the alpha granules are the most abundant and have an important role in regenerative and wound healing processes [4–6]. They contain adhesive proteins, growth factors, and clot-forming factors. The regenerative function of the alpha granules is based on mitogenic factors such as vascular endothelial growth factor (VEGF), platelet-derived growth factor (PDGF), fibroblast growth factor (FGF), epidermal growth factor (EGF), hepatocyte growth factor (HGF), and insulin-like growth factor (IGF)) [5–7].

In order for the granule release from a cell to occur, platelet activation is required. This process is mediated by platelet activating molecules and some of these molecules are produced by platelets (e.g., collagen, thrombin, thromboxane A, adenosine phosphate, P-selectin, and protease activator receptor–related molecules). On contrary, there are so-called inhibitors that act as platelet receptors' inhibiting molecules, thereby preventing platelet activation (e.g., coagulation factors, aspirin, ADP receptor inhibitors).

Once a blood vessel is injured and there is a rupture at the level of the endothelial layer, platelets start releasing molecules, such as collagen, that activate them. Activated platelets bind to the injured site of the blood vessel with collagen. This is known as adhesion. In addition, activated platelets secrete great amounts of ADP and, at the same time, thromboxane A2 is being synthesized, which then initiates granule (alpha and dense) release, which, in return, results in platelet aggregation. In other words, white platelet clot formation, that is, a result of the processes we explained beforehand, has three stages: platelet adhesion, granule release, and platelet aggregation. Simultaneously with platelet activation, blood vessel injury initiates a coagulation cascade. It starts when blood interacts with tissue factors. This process entails a series of biochemical reactions that convert inactive blood plasma proteins to active proteolytic enzymes. In this way, the coagulation process—that starts with thrombin activation upon blood vessel injury—ends with the conversion of fibrinogen to fibrin. As a result, fibrin fibers permeate and secure the thrombus. In this way, the process of hemostasis is accomplished [4, 5, 7].

3. Platelet concentrates

Platelets are not limited to hemostatic processes, but they also influence tissue regeneration, enhance collagen synthesis, and trigger angiogenesis as well as the immune response by releasing growth factors and cytokines [6]. The concept of platelet concentrate preparation is based on the fact that manipulation of normal physiologic processes, such as hemostasis, enables us to obtain concentrated platelets together with a greater amount of growth factors that play a crucial role in wound healing. They do that by stimulating tissue regeneration and proliferation, initiating extracellular matrix deposition, and supporting cell differentiation. By obtaining platelet concentrates, we obtain autologous biomaterials that have an important role in regenerative procedures. To date, there are numerous patents related to platelet concentrates [6]. The first one to be invented was, however, the fibrin glue, and it serves as the precursor of platelet concentrates afterward. Later, PRF (platelet-rich fibrin), sticky bone, and plasma gel were invented. The preparation process is simple. In outline, it is required to draw an adequate amount of blood from a patient in vacuum test tubes with or without anticoagulants and centrifuge them according to a protocol of choice. The point is that with every novel method of platelet concentrate preparation, scientists have struggled to improve the earlier one. The main objective was to increase the number of growth factors and prolong their release time. Novel methods made easier the preparation process by eliminating anticoagulants and simplifying centrifuge protocols.

Further in this chapter, we discuss a brief review of the most important platelet concentrates.

3.1 Fibrin glue

The fibrin glue is a precursor to platelet concentrates, application of which in medicine started 50 years ago. It is packed in two bottles with different content. One bottle contains lyophilized human fibrinogen, while another one contains either bovine or human thrombin. The mandatory ingredients are calcium salts. Proper usage entails mixing the contents of the two bottles, whereby the coagulation process is imitated, and a gel-like formulation is formed (fibrin clot) that can further be used as a topical hemostatic, tissue adhesive (glue), as well as to join bone graft particles. Although they do have broad applications, fibrin glues have several disadvantages, among which is costly manufacture that makes them less popular in comparison to platelet concentrates [6].

3.2 Platelet-rich plasma

Platelet-rich plasma (PRP) belongs to the first generation of platelet concentrates that were put into practice by Robert Marx in 1998. PRP is an autologous human platelet concentrate in a small plasma volume. Precisely, it consists of 1 million platelets per 1 microliter in a total volume of 5 milliliters of plasma. Platelet activation in PRP leads to a release of a variety of growth factors that have an important role in the regulation and stimulation of healing.

The PRP preparation process can be divided into the following phases (**Figure 1**):

- Blood drawing into vacuum test tubes with the anticoagulant (3.2% sodium citrate)
- First centrifugation with the relative centrifugation force (rcf) of 200 g for 10 minutes

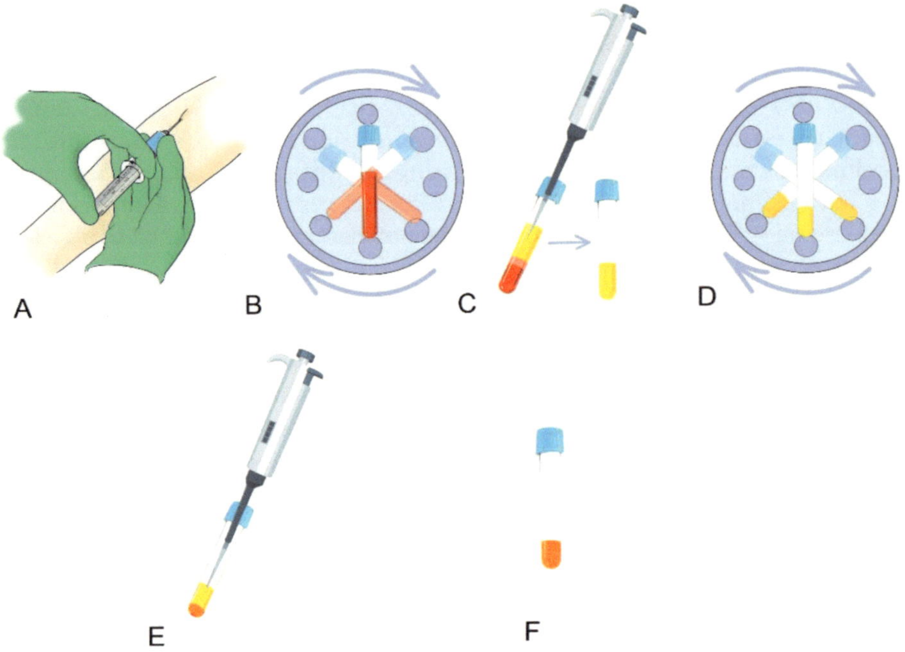

Figure 1.
The PRP preparation process. (A) Blood drawing into 3.2% sodium citrate vacuum test tubes. (B) First centrifugation. (C) Transferring the supernatant to a sterile test tube. (D) Second centrifugation. (E) Removal of two-thirds of the supernatant (PPP). (F) Final product platelet-rich plasma (PRP).

- Transferring the supernatant to a sterile test tube and performing the second centrifugation at 2500 g for 15 minutes
- Upon completion of the second centrifugation, removal of two-thirds of the supernatant should be performed as it represents the platelet-poor plasma (PPP)
- The rest should be gently shaken to obtain the PRP.

When prepared accordingly, the PRP is in a liquid state due to the anticoagulant presence and can be stored for up to 8 hours in sterile conditions. Before using the PRP, calcium chloride and bovine thrombin should be added, thereby activating platelets that trigger coagulation processes, which, in return, results in a PRP transition from liquid to gel-like state. Activated thrombocytes release the granules—growth factors and cytokines.

Activated growth factors interact with the cell membrane. They never enter the cell or the nucleus. Consequently, they do not have a mutagenic potential; rather, they stimulate physiological healing processes only [8–10].

When in a liquid state, PRP can be injected into a tissue, or it can be mixed with biomaterials that serve as a substitute for bone. In contact with tissue collagen, platelet activation ensues. Activated PRP transitions to a gel, so it can be used as a membrane, or it can be mixed with bone grafts to obtain a graft with a specific shape.

A disadvantage to PRP is a complicated preparation as well as the presence of foreign substances such as anticoagulants (sodium citrate) and procoagulants (calcium chloride and bovine thrombin). Each of these substances can have an antigenic effect albeit, according to Marx, bovine thrombin does not have any contact with systemic circulation and is used in small quantities.

3.3 Platelet rich in growth factors (PRGF)

Platelet-rich growth factors were first described in 1999 by Eduardo Anitua, who patented PRGF within Biotechnology Institute, BTI, Vitoria, Spain, a dental implant company. For PRGF to be made, it requires one centrifugation only coupled by multiple pipetting to ensure precise isolation of the centrifugation end-products. The result is a preparation rich in growth factors, however, with no leukocytes [10, 11].

The procedure requires the following equipment: PRGF system centrifuge, four calibrated test tubes with anticoagulants, Plasmatherm (heating device), micropipettes, and activator (calcium chloride). The preparation phases are the following (**Figure 2**):

- Drawing of 9 ml of patient's blood in vacuum test tubes with anticoagulant (sodium citrate).
- Centrifugation in the PRGF system centrifuge at the rcf of 460 g for 8 minutes.
- At the end of the centrifugation, two layers can be seen: yellow (top) and red (bottom). The top yellow layer is composed of three fractions (top to bottom).
- Fraction 1 has a volume of 1 ml and is used for fibrine membrane preparation. This fraction is growth factor poor, hence the name: platelet poor in growth factors (PPGF).
- Fraction 2 has a volume of 0.5 ml and contains growth factors, hence the name: plasma with growth factors (PGF).
- Fraction 3 has a volume of 0.5 ml and represents plasma rich in growth factors (PRGF).
- Bellow Fraction 3 there is a thin layer of leukocytes that is not utilized.

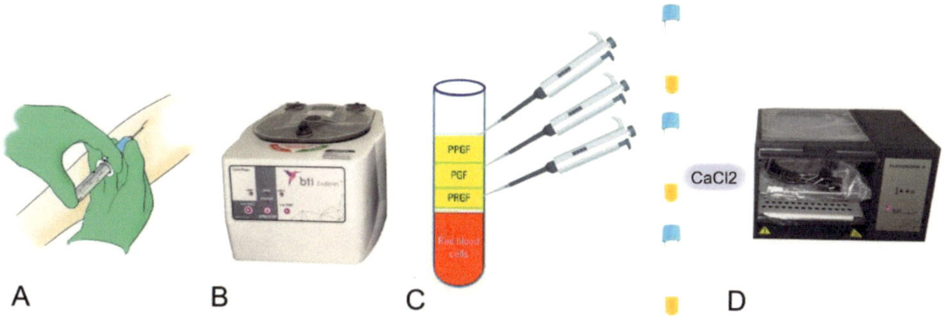

Figure 2.
The PRGF preparation process. (A) Blood drawing into 3.2% sodium citrate vacuum test tubes. (B) BTI centrifuge (PRGF system centrifuge. (C) Micropipetting PPGF, PGF, and PRGF fractions. (D) Three fractions transferred into calibrated tubes and activated with $CaCl_2$ and heating device (Plasmatherm).

PRGF prepared in this way is activated by procoagulant calcium chloride, whereby 50 μl of calcium chloride is used in 1 ml of PRGF. It takes 6 minutes for PRGF to transition from a liquid to a gel-like state upon activation and, as such, it becomes an autologous biomaterial ready for use. Plasmatherm (a device used for heating) should be set at 37°C to accelerate the transition.

In contrast to the previous, this protocol requires one centrifugation only. Instead of using bovine thrombin, it requires using calcium chloride to activate coagulation, while coagulation acceleration is achieved by using Plasmatherm. The greatest difference between PRGF and other platelet concentrates is the absence of leukocytes in the final product that is used as a biomaterial. Anitua et al., however, consider this as an advantage as they argue that proinflammatory activity is thereby prevented. This question remains controversial since there are many conflicting opinions among scientists.

3.4 Platelet-rich fibrin (PRF)

Platelet-rich fibrin belongs to the second generation of platelet concentrates. It was patented by Joseph Choukroun in 2000. In contrast to the previous platelet concentrates, this one does not require the use of anticoagulants or bovine thrombin as procoagulants. The principle behind preparing this autologous biomaterial starts with physiologically triggered coagulation processes. The equipment required is a phlebotomy pack, vacuum test tubes, and a centrifuge with a fixed angle [12].

The authentic PRF protocol is the leukocyte (L-PRF) or Choukroun's protocol (**Figure 3**), which contains the phases listed below:

- Drawing patient's blood in 9–10 ml volumed vacuum test tubes without anticoagulants
- Prompt transport of the blood to the centrifuge is required followed by centrifugation at 2700 rpm for 12 minutes.

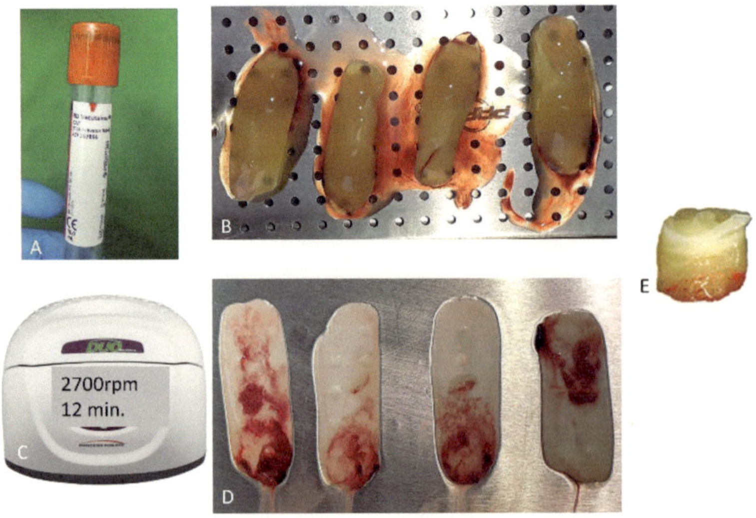

Figure 3.
L-PRF protocol. (A) Vacutainer with clot activator. (B) PRF clots. (C) Centrifuge with chosen protocol. (D) PRF membranes. (E) PRF plug.

- After some time, platelets that come in contact with the sidewalls of test tubes become activated. This is when the coagulation starts.

- Fibrinogen, initially concentrated at the top of the test tube, is mixed with circulating thrombin and then transformed into fibrin. In this way, the fibrin clot, located in the middle of the test tube, is formed.

- There can be visualized two distinct layers in the test tube upon centrifugation: yellow (top) and red (bottom). There is acellular plasma at the top of the yellow layer, while below that, there is a fibrin clot or so-called PRF.

- It is a rule of thumb that test tubes are placed in a test tube holder after centrifugation is done. Also, the test tubes should be left open for 5 minutes for the clots to mature.

- The matured clots are then extrapolated from the test tubes and placed on the grid of the PRF box. A lid should then be placed on the top of the clots to serve as a weight for the remaining liquid to exit the clots. Such clots are then turned into membranes, hence the name: PRF membranes.

Apart from the PRF membranes, PRF plugs can also be made from the PRF clots. For this purpose, PRF clots need to be put into cylinders of the PRF box. On the top, stainless steel weights need to be placed to eliminate the residual liquid. By using this approach, clots are turned into plugs or disks of desired height.

PRF clots contain 100% platelets and the growth factors from the patient's blood sample. Additionally, they contain 65% leukocytes, which are the growth factor source, especially for PDGF and VEGF.

Besides platelets and leukocytes, PRF contains fibrin too.

There are multiple roles of fibrin in PRF:

- Stimulates angiogenesis—supports microvascularization

- Supports the immune system

- Covers wounds, stimulates epithelization, and enhances healing

- Helps leukocyte migration—a significant role in infected wounds

PRF membrane and PRF disks or plugs are also called solid PRF.

Numerous protocols have been invented to obtain advanced PRF forms. Most of them are based on the change in velocity and time required for centrifugation. The objective was to obtain PRF with the best characteristics possible—uniform platelet distribution along the clot and prolonged growth factor release.

In the text below, we will further be discussing different types of PRF.

3.4.1 Leukocyte-platelet-rich fibrin (L-PRF)

L-PRF is the original version of solid PRF. It was first prepared by centrifuging samples at rcf of 400 g for 12 minutes [13]. The end product was a PRF clot that was used for PRF membrane and plug preparation. The research has shown that the majority of the growth factors could be found at the bottom of a membrane or plug rather than them being evenly distributed across the structures. This can also be considered a disadvantage of L-PRF.

3.4.2 Advanced platelet-rich fibrin (A-PRF)

Advanced platelet-rich fibrin came to light in 2014 [14]. It was a result of a newly introduced slow centrifugation concept, objective of which was to prevent cell loss and increase the number of viable cells. A-PRF has a greater number of leukocytes, platelets, neutrophils, and lymphocytes and has been suggested to have a prolonged growth factor release [13]. It is obtained by centrifuging samples at the rcf of 208 g for 14 minutes [13]. In comparison to the L-PRF membrane, the A-PRF membrane is shorter, has a greater cell-retaining capacity, and it releases larger amounts of growth factors [9, 15].

3.4.3 Advanced A-PRF+

A-PRF+ is a variant of the A-PRF obtained by decreasing the time needed to centrifuge samples while remaining a constant relative centrifugation force of 208 g. Instead of centrifuging samples for 14 minutes, this protocol requires one to do so for 8 minutes [16]. In comparison with the A-PRF and L-PRF, A-PRF+ has been shown to release even greater amounts of growth factors, especially TGF-β1, VEGF, PDGF, EGF, and IGF1 [13, 17].

3.4.4 Advanced liquid PRF (A-PRF liquid)

A-PRF liquid can be prepared by centrifuging samples at 1300 rpm for 5 minutes. The end-product is in a liquid state, which allows it to be mixed with bone grafts, whereby so-called sticky bone is obtained. It can also be used for large membrane preparation.

3.4.5 Injectable PRF (i-PRF)

Injectable PRF is a liquid form of PRF intended for a variety of purposes including but not limited to tissue injections, mixing with grafts to obtain sticky bone, skin injections in the facial region to achieve rejuvenation, joint injections, and large membrane preparation. Choukroun has patented several types of i-PRF:

3.4.5.1 i-PRF

i-PRF can be considered a universal protocol for injectable PRF. The protocol instructs blood sample centrifugation at 700 rpm for 3 minutes.

3.4.5.2 i-PRF M

This protocol is intended for males since they naturally have a greater number of erythrocytes. Consequently, the centrifugation time needs to be longer compared to protocols addressing i-PRF preparation for women to ensure larger quantities of centrifuged i-PRF. In short, it should be centrifuged at 700 rpm for 4 minutes.

3.4.5.3 i-PRF+

The i-PRF+ protocol requires centrifuging blood samples at 700 rpm for 5 minutes. Its purpose lies in obtaining a liquid PRF that is oftentimes used for facial esthetic procedures as well as in orthopedic surgeries.

A novel protocol introduced in 2019 (1300 rpm for 14 minutes) by Choukroun covered both solid and liquid PRF preparation and simplified the preparation process. Namely, this protocol allows us to place test tubes for solid (A-PRF) and liquid PRF (S-PRF, i-PRF+) immediately upon taking blood samples in the very same centrifuge and spinning them according to the same protocol. Consequently, this protocol amnesties us from using different protocols for solid and liquid PRF preparation.

3.5 Sacco's protocol for obtaining concentrated growth factors in solid form (CGF) and concentrated growth factors in liquid form (LPCGF)

Sacco's concept entails three major steps. The first is acceleration whereby samples are accelerated for 30 seconds from 0 to 2700 rpm. This is followed by a combination of four protocols (2 minutes 2700 rpm, 4 minutes 2400 rpm, 4 minutes 2700 rpm, and 3 minutes 3000 rpm). Lastly, samples are deaccelerated for 36 seconds (from 3000 rpm to 0). The difference between CGF and LPCGF is in the type of test tubes used. Solid CGF uses glass red cap tubes (PV 200R—Medifuge Blood Separator CGF P Cycle), while liquid LPCGF uses the red cap tubes (PV 200R) with added sodium heparin or blue cap tubes (PV 200P) with separator gel and sodium citrate (Medifuge Blood Separator CGF Cycle) [18–20].

3.6 BIO-PRF

BIO-PRF was introduced to the practice by Richard J Miron. In contrast to Choukroun's concept, which uses a fixed centrifugation angle, Richard's concept uses horizontal centrifugation [21]. This centrifugation method has already been known and has been in use for PRP production; however, it is only after the BIO-PRF protocol had been introduced that it became commercially available for PRF production. This is because the BIO-PRF protocol mandates the usage of horizontal centrifuge [21].

The advantage of horizontal centrifugation lies in the benefit of attaining greater platelet and leukocyte concentrations in both solid and liquid states of PRF. These cells are more evenly distributed across the PRF clot [21]. The concentration of released growth factors is greater. There is less cellular damage and the accumulation of erythrocytes on the sidewalls of test tubes is rare [21].

Miron's BIO-PRF concept we use today encompasses four protocols:

- Solid PRF
- Liquid PRF
- C PRF
- ALB-PRF

3.6.1 Solid PRF

Solid PRF is prepared by horizontally centrifuging samples at rcf of 700 g for 8 minutes. This protocol is used for PRF membrane preparation from PRF clots.

3.6.2 Liquid PRF

Liquid PRF is also prepared by horizontally centrifuging samples at rcf of 300 g for 5 minutes. This method enables us to attain greater concentrations of both leukocytes and platelets.

3.6.3 C PRF

C PRF is a concentrated PRF, hence its acronym. It is prepared by using a strong centrifugal force of 2000 g for 8 minutes. The result is a greater concentration of platelets, leukocytes, and monocytes in the so-called buffy coat, immediately above the red layer, in which volume ranges from 0.3 to 0.5 mL [22].

The difference between C PRF and i-PRF is in the concentration of platelets; C PRF has a 15 times greater concentration of platelets, while i-PRF has only 2–3 times greater concentration. A very similar situation can be found with leukocytes whose concentrations can be even 500% greater [22].

3.6.4. ALB-PRF (autologous albumin gel and liquid platelet-rich fibrin)

ALB-PRF was made to prolong the regenerative potential of a classical PRF membrane. Namely, the issue is that the PRF membrane becomes resorbed after 15 days at most. Consequently, its regenerative potential, that is, growth factors release, ceases. Due to fast resorption, PRF membranes are not applicable as independent barrier membranes for procedures such as GBR (guide bone regeneration) and GTR (guide tissue regeneration).

The idea to use heat for prolonging PRF membrane viability was introduced by Kawase et al. in 2015. In contrast to classical PRF membranes, Kawase's heat-compressed PRF was visible even 3 weeks after an in vivo implantation [23]. Although the thermally processed PRF/PPP has had longer viability, its regenerative potential was compromised considering that no cell or growth factor molecule could survive undergoing processes of denaturation (thermal heating) [24]. This has motivated Mour et al. to modify the production protocol of a membrane that consists of a combination of concentrated growth factors and denaturized albumin gel (ALB-CGF) [20]. The protocol entails drawing 9 ml of blood into plastic test tubes without anticoagulants and other additives. This is followed by a centrifugation process according to the protocol for concentrated growth factors in a liquid state by using Medifuge (Silfradent) centrifuge (acceleration for 30 seconds from 0 to 2700 rpm then combination of 4 protocols: 2700 rpm for 2 minutes, 2400 rpm for 4 minutes, 2700 rpm for 4 minutes, 3000 rpm for 3 minutes followed by deacceleration that should last 36 seconds) [20]. The yellow top layer, formed upon centrifugation, consists of platelet-poor plasma (PPP) that can be collected by a syringe in a volume of 2 ml, liquid phase concentrated growth factors (LPCGF), and buffy coat that can also be collected by a syringe in a volume of 4 ml [20]. The PPP in the syringe is then transferred to a special machine that increases its temperature to 75°C for 10 minutes. The heating process leads toward albumin denaturation and albumin gel formation. This is then left in a sterile glass container. Once the gel has cooled down, LPCGF and a buffy coat are poured upon it. It takes 5 minutes for polymerization to finish after which the ALB-CGF membrane, the end-product, is obtained. It has a usage potential in guide tissue regeneration because it resorbs after 4–6 months [20, 24]. However, researchers could not prove that the ALB-CGF membrane can release growth factors in a prolonged manner [20].

Modernized protocol for ALB-PRF membrane consists of the following steps [24]:

- Drawing 9 ml of blood into plastic test tubes without anticoagulants and other additives
- Horizontal centrifugation by using Bio-PRF centrifuge at 700 g for 8 minutes. In this way, the top yellow layer becomes divided layers: the top
- Layer that is platelet-poor, and the bottom layer, which is platelet- and growth factor-rich.
- Use a syringe to evacuate 2 ml of PPP from the top by using an 18G needle
- Put a cap on a syringe and place it in the middle portion of the heating machine (Bio-Heat). The heating (75°C) should last for 10 minutes
- Test tubes with the residual liquid PRF should be kept in the Bio-Cool device to prevent clotting
- After heating the syringe with albumin gel, it should be cooled down in the Bio-Cool device for 1–2 minutes
- Cool ALB gel from the syringe should be poured into a container and shaped
- Use a syringe to evacuate the remaining 1–2 mL of C-PRF (buffy coat) and pour it over the ALB gel. It is required to wait for 15 minutes before usage
- The end product is an ALB-PRF membrane with improved characteristics (**Figure 4**).

Upcoming clinical studies will provide us with more benefits concerning the ALB PRF membrane.

3.7 Sticky bone (concentrated growth factors enriched bone graft matrix)

Sticky bone is a mixture of autologous fibrin glue and bone grafts (autografts, xenografts, allografts) [25]. Sticky bone is also known as a mineralized plasmatic matrix [26–38]. A bone graft obtained in this way is gelatinous in structure, which renders it for shaping. It is rich in growth factors, thereby accelerating tissue regeneration [39, 40]. It has many indications in oral and periodontal surgery as well as in implantology.

Sticky bone can be prepared by using PRP, PRGF, and i-PRF. All these formulations are in a liquid state and are prepared according to different protocols. They differ in their activation mechanisms—transformation to activated platelet gel. To summarize, when in a liquid state, they mix with bone particles or grafts and upon activation they transform to a gel-like state, hence leaving us with a gelatinous mass that we can further shape.

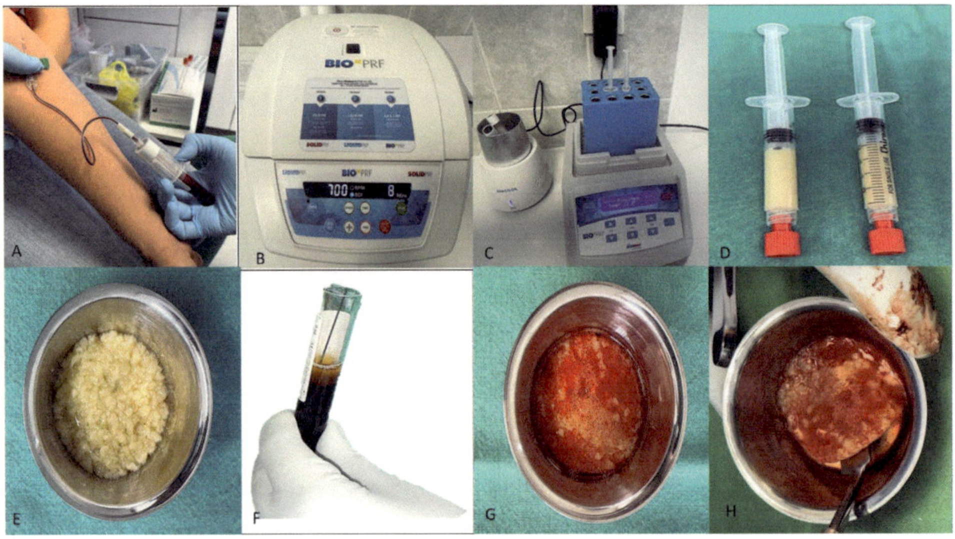

Figure 4.
Modernized ALB-PRF protocol. (A) Blood sampling into PET tubes. (B) BIO-PRF centrifuge set on rcf of 700 g for 8 min. (C) Bio-Cool and Bio-Heat device. (D) Syringes with ALB-gel. (E) ALB-gel in a bowl. (F) C-PRF-buffy coat. (G) Immediately after pouring C-PRF into cooled ALB-gel. (H) ALB-PRF membrane.

3.7.1 Different sticky bone preparation protocols

3.7.1.1 Sticky bone with PRP

This method entails PRP preparation according to the already established protocol. This is followed by mixing PRP with bone graft. For the mixture to become gelatinous, it should be activated by thrombin of a bovine origin or from autogenic serum. To enhance this, calcium chloride can be added as well.

3.7.1.2 Sticky bone with PRGF

PRGF obtained according to the established protocol is mixed with a bone graft. The mixture is then activated by adding calcium chloride and heating.

3.7.1.3 Sticky bone with i-PRF

This method has two main advantages:

- It uses test tubes without anticoagulants for PRF preparation
- The protocol for i-PRF is simplified (only one centrifugation is required according to either Choukroun's or Miron's protocol for liquid PRF preparation).

To prepare sticky bone, already prepared i-PRF is mixed with a bone graft. Thanks to physiologic coagulation processes, the mixture becomes gelatinous after some time. To accelerate the coagulation process and to enhance density and firmness, adding 1–2 fibrin clots to the mixture can be considered (**Figure 5**).

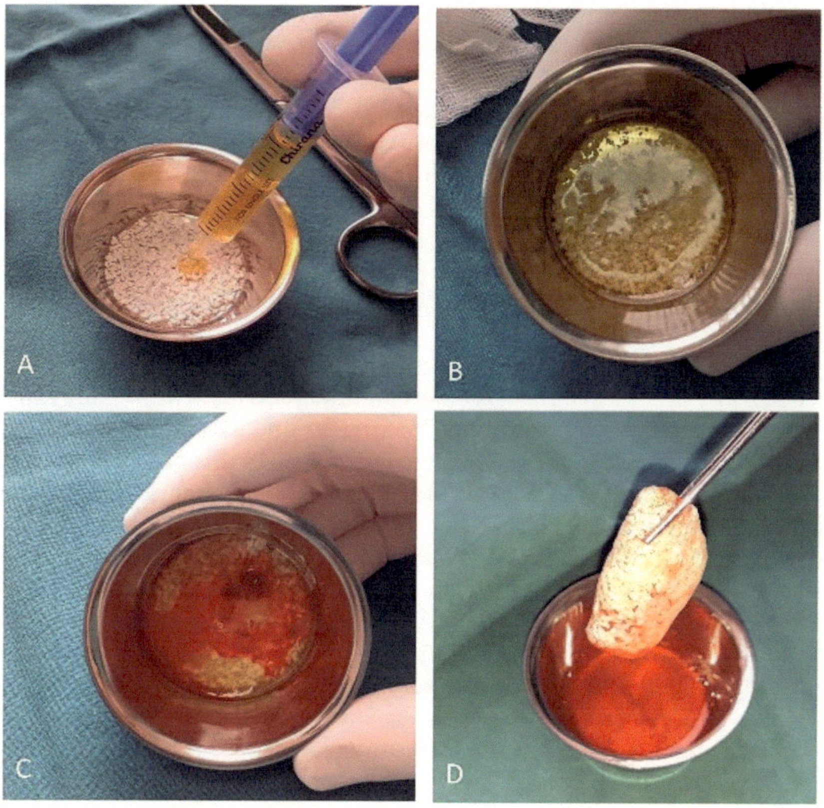

Figure 5.
Making sticky bone. A) Adding i-PRF into the bone substitute. B) Gel starting to form. C) Gelling completed. D) Sticky bone.

Sticky bone can be also prepared in a way that uses scissors to cut one or two PRF membranes into pieces. This is followed by adding a required amount of bone graft, thereby making a mixture. This should be thoroughly mixed all together with a PRF exudate. The PRF exudate is a liquid that is segregated upon PRF clot compression in the process of PRF membrane preparation. It contains autologous thrombin that stimulates coagulation as well as gelatinization. This gel-like mass can further be shaped in the desired shape. Every few seconds, i-PRF should be added to it drop by drop. In several minutes, the mass becomes gelatinous, and the sticky bone formed in this is ready for use.

3.8 BIO-bone

Bio-bone is a variant of sticky bone. It has improved characteristics and was patented by Richard Miron. Bio-bone is, in fact, a combination of Alb-gel, bone graft, and injectable PRF. In other words, in this autologous biomaterial, bone graft and ALB-PRF membrane with prolonged viability (4–6 months) are found together.

A Bio-PRF preparation protocol is identical to the ALB-PRF membrane preparation protocol. However, there is one distinction: after pouring one part of a liquid PRF (CGF) over a cooled ALB-gel, a layer of bone graft (preferably allograft) should be added to it. Furthermore, the rest of the PRF (CGF) should be poured over this construction. It takes 15 minutes for this mass to become gelatinous and ready for use.

Thanks to the prolonged viability of the ALB-PRF membrane, sticky bone prepared in this way can be used in augmentative procedures without the usage of a collagenous membrane, consequently reducing the financial costs of the procedure.

4. PRF preparation equipment

4.1 Centrifuge

The concept of PRF preparation is based on full blood centrifugation, which results in blood components' separation (for simpler understanding: red and yellow fractions). Relative centrifugation force (rcf) is the key in this process rather than rotations per minute (rpm) that represents a variable parameter dependable on centrifuge design and radius [41].

Nowadays, there are different protocols for PRF preparation that use centrifuges with different rotors, test tube angulation and design [42]. These protocols are based on the rpm values rather than rcf values. Although there are numerous articles addressing PRF, they cannot be adequately compared simply due to the heterogeneity in rcf reporting [41]. In other words, the very same protocol that utilizes different centrifuges provides us with different results. For this reason, it is highly important to use certified centrifuges such as the Intraspin device for L-PRF protocol (that has a fixed centrifuge angle of 33°), Duo Quatro centrifuge for A-PRF+ protocol (that has a fixed centrifuge angle of 40°), and Bio-PRF centrifuge for Bio-PRF protocol (that has horizontal centrifugation adjustment) (**Figure 6**) [42].

4.2 Vacuum test tubes for platelet concentrate preparation procedures

In the process of obtaining platelet concentrates, vacuum test tubes (also known as vacutainer tubes) are used. There are two types of test tubes: glass- and plastic-made test tubes (**Figure 7**).

The advantage of using glass test tubes lies in the glass' ability to stimulate coagulation [43]. Considering that a modern approach to PRF preparation entails the avoidance of additives and anticoagulants, empty glass test tubes are the ideal choice for PRF membrane and plug preparation. In case we opt for plastic test tubes, they should be equipped with a clot activator that accelerates the coagulation process. Such activators are micronized silica particles that coat the inside surface of vacutainers. If a test tube is coated with a clot activator, then its wall is blurred. Regardless of that, it has recently been reported that silica particles have side effect [44]. It is mostly related to a possible negative effect on tissue regeneration, cytotoxic effect, cell apoptosis, and PRF clot size [44–46]. Albeit no serious side effects have been reported up to date, it is recommended to use test tubes without any chemical additives [44–46].

Plastic vacuum test tubes without additives are made of polyethylene terephthalate (PET) plastic [47]. In contrast to glass and silica particle-coated plastic test tubes with a red cap that are hydrophile, these plastic test tubes are hydrophobic. In these test tubes, the yellow fraction (liquid PRF) remains in a liquid state for 30 minutes under the hermetic conditions upon centrifugation. In conclusion, these test tubes are used

DOI: http://dx.doi.org/10.5772/intechopen.108807

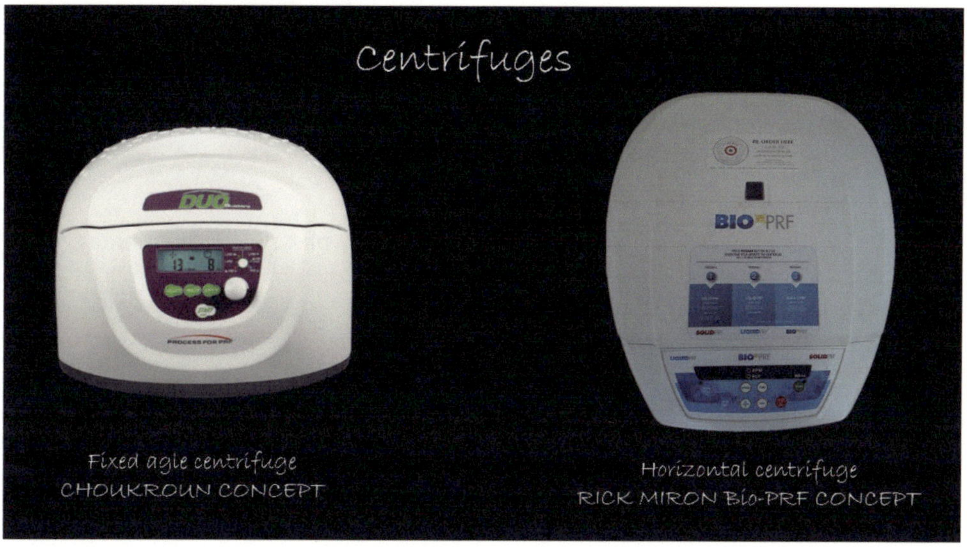

Figure 6.
Fixed angle and horizontal centrifuge.

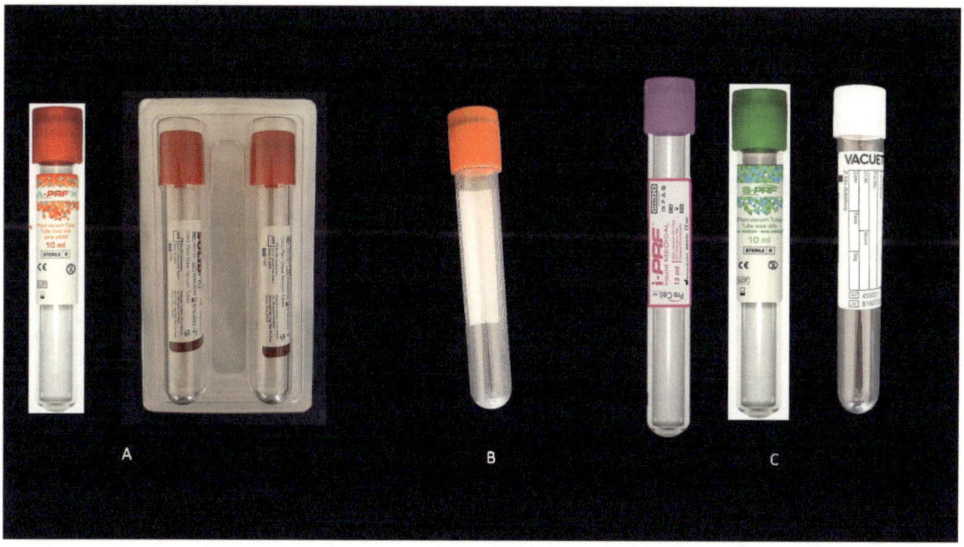

Figure 7.
Blood collection tubes. (A) 10 ml glass vacuum red cap tubes for PRF membranes. (B) 10 ml silica-coated plastic tube with no additive for PRF membranes. (C) 13 ml, 10 ml, and 9 ml PET tubes with no additive added for sticky bone, large PRF membranes, and facial esthetics.

in liquid PRF, CGF, and sticky bone preparation. Liquid PRF nowadays is frequently used in facial esthetic procedures.

A correct test tube selection is of vital importance for obtaining safe and high-quality PRF products. Oftentimes this may be an issue considering that there are test tubes of low and ambiguous quality in the market. For this reason, clinicians are recommended to use test tubes from safe and trustworthy retailers.

4.3 Phlebotomy equipment

Phlebotomy equipment includes Esmarch's tourniquet and blood collection butterfly needles with tube holders (**Figure 8**).

4.4 PRF kit

Besides an appropriate centrifuge and test tubes, the basic PRF kit includes (**Figure 9**):

- Test tube holder
- PRF box (for PRF membrane and plug production)
- PRF hand tools (bone compactors, double-ended graft spoon, PRF pad, PRF forceps, scissors).

5. Examples of PRF and sticky bone applications in oral surgery

There are many indications for PRF and sticky bone usage in dentistry. In this section, only indications related to oral surgery and implantology will be discussed further.

5.1 Immediate dental implant placement after tooth extraction: single-phase approach

If the extraction of a multi-rooted tooth was atraumatic—that is, with preservation of the interradicular septum—it is possible to place an implant altogether with empty alveoli augmentation. An example is shown in **Figure 10**. In this patient, there was an indication to extract the first mandibular molar tooth. Immediately after the atraumatic extraction, an implant was placed in the intact

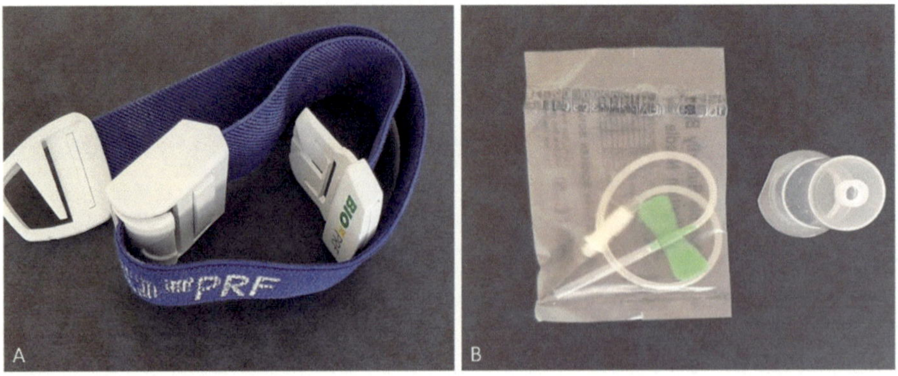

Figure 8.
Phlebotomy equipment. (A) Esmarch's tourniquet. (B) Safety butterfly blood collection needle with holder.

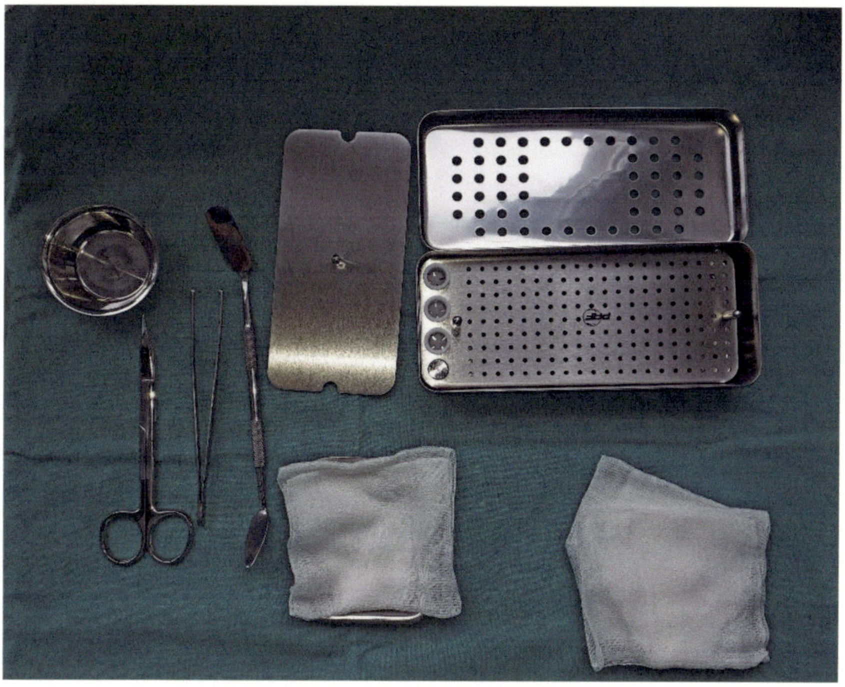

Figure 9.
Basic PRF kit.

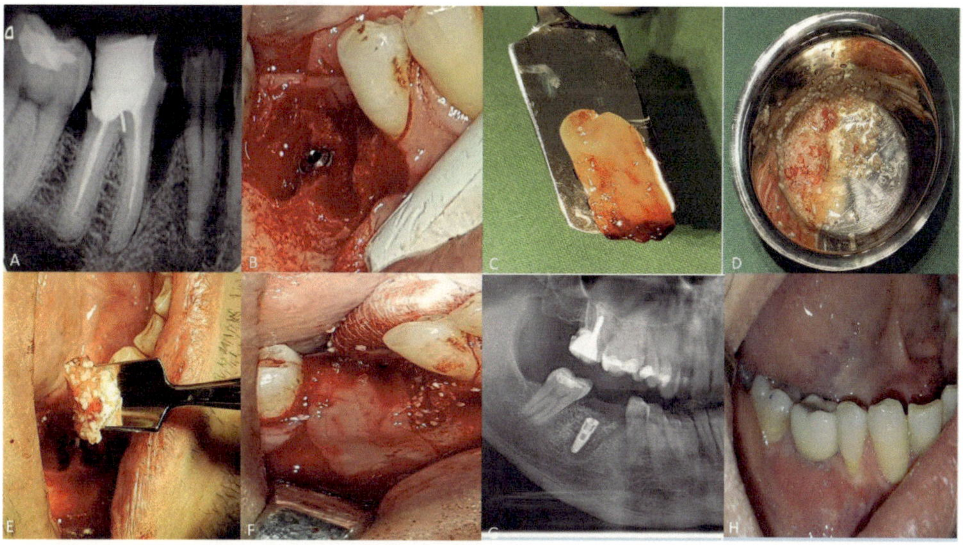

Figure 10.
Implant placement immediately after tooth extraction. (A) Tooth indicated for extraction. (B) Implant placed into inter-radicular septum. (C) PRF membrane. (D) A mixture of PRF membrane cut into pieces and bone substitute. (E) Grafting the empty alveolar socket. (F) PRF membranes adapted over graft. (G) OPG view of inserted implant (H) final prosthetics—screw-retained crown.

interradicular septum. The empty alveoli were augmented by a mixture of bone graft and PRF membrane pieces. As a bone replacement, Novocor plus bone was used. It is a natural bone grafting material consisting of natural coral granules—Madreporic Coral consisting of 98% aragonite calcium carbonate. A PRF membrane covering the structure was placed. This was followed by positioning of the apical mattress stitch and a primary suturing of the elongated flap. After an osteointegration period, the patient was readmitted for a prosthetic procedure that entailed screw-retained crown placement.

5.2 Implant placement after tooth extraction and residual alveolar ridge augmentation: two-phase approach

This example (**Figure 11**) represents a case of a patient with severe periodontitis (horizontal and vertical bone loss) affecting two molar teeth. In the first visit, extraction of the two molar teeth ensued followed by a thorough curettage. Additionally, bone augmentation with sticky bone was performed. As a bone graft, Novocor plus bone was used. Nine months later, one implant was placed in the augmented region.

5.3 Single implant placement in lower jaw with an insufficient vertical and horizontal dimension

This case is presenting immediate implant placement in the lower jaw in the premolar region with a lack of bone height and width. The patient had complicated extraction of root 44, which led to greater bone loss. Implant placement was carefully planned with the help of a 3D CBCT scan. Since there was a lack of bone height

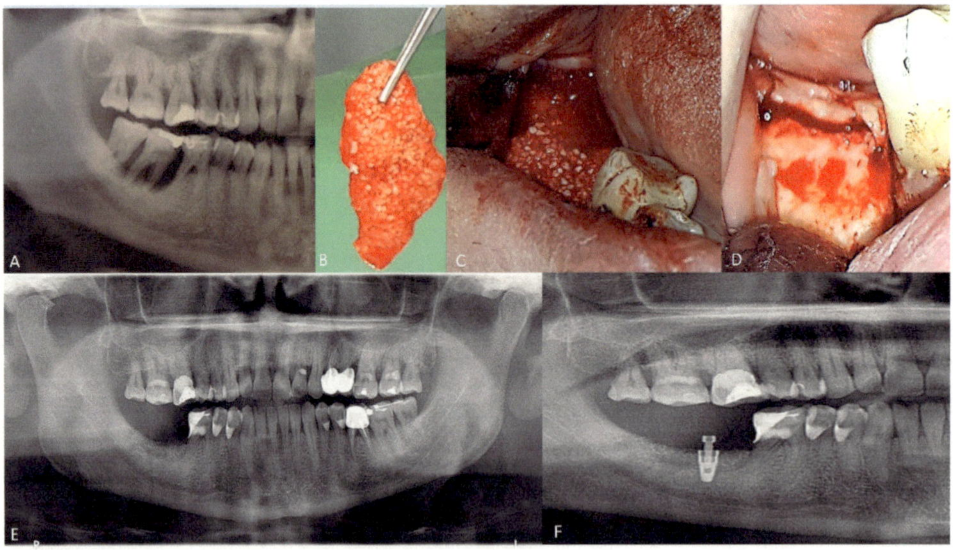

Figure 11.
Implant placement 9 months after bone augmentation- two-phase approach. (A) Teeth 47 and 48 indicated for extraction. (B) Sticky bone. (C) Grafted area. (D) Clinical appearance 9 months after augmentation with sticky bone. (E) OPG view 9 months after augmentation with sticky bone. (F) OPG of the implant inserted into the augmented bone.

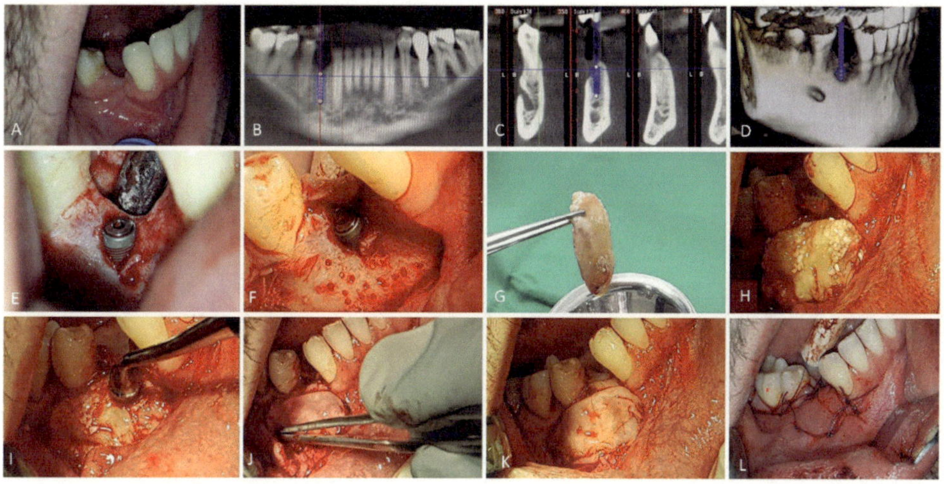

Figure 12.
Single implant placement in lower jaw with an insufficient vertical and horizontal dimension. (A) Clinical appearance of the area where the implant should be inserted. (B–D) CBCT planning. (E and F) The implant threads are exposed. (G) Sticky bone. (H–J) Augmentation with sticky bone. (L) Flap repositioned and sutured.

toward the mental canal, we planned to leave part of the implant not covered by bone and above the crest line. Missing bone was augmented with the help of artificial bone Novocor plus in combination with platelet-rich fibrin creating "sticky bone." The implant used in this case was 3P by BB dental, and later we placed a screw-retained metal-ceramic crown (**Figure 12**).

5.4 Lateral sinus lift with sticky bone coupled with a simultaneous implant placement

Tooth loss results in bone resorption. In the transcanine sector of the maxilla, the most characteristic consequence of tooth loss is the lowering of the maxillary sinus, which imposes unfavorable conditions for implant placement. In the cases when the indication for implant placement exists, whereby the height of the remaining bone is less than 5 mm, a lateral sinus lift procedure is done. In this example (**Figure 13**), lateral sinus lift with sticky bone and PRF membrane usage coupled with three dental implant placements was done in a single visit. At the end of the osteointegration process, which went without any complications, three single screw-retained crowns were placed.

5.5 Apicoectomy with a huge cystectomy in the maxilla

This case (**Figure 14**) represents a huge radicular maxillary cyst encompassing three teeth (11, 21, and 22). The cyst has destroyed a part of the vestibular and palatine bone with its expansive growth. Once endodontic treatment of the affected teeth had been done, apicoectomy with cystectomy was performed. The bony defect was filled with a sticky bone, which was prepared with a xenograft (BioSS). This was covered with PRF membranes and a collagen membrane. The flap was repositioned and sutured. Three months after the surgery, the OPG X-Ray (**Figure 12L**) shows excellent signs of bone regeneration.

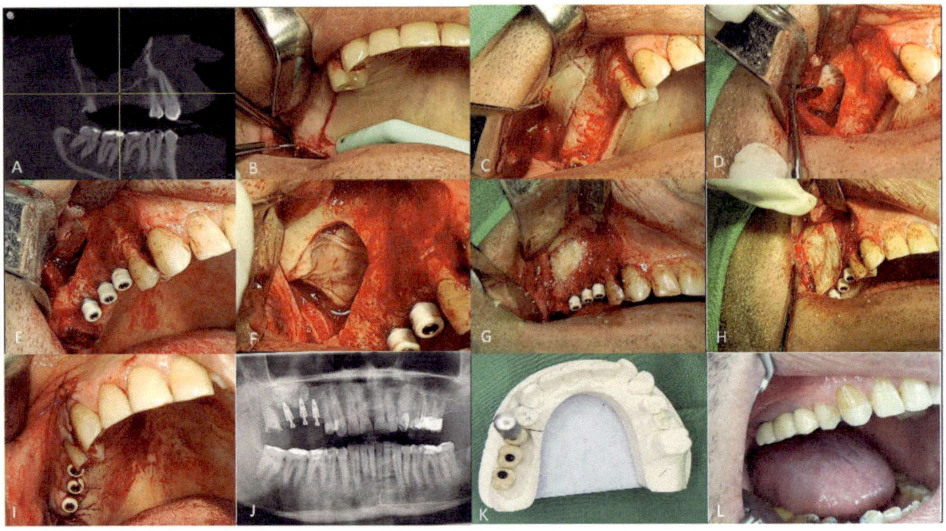

Figure 13.
(A) Insufficient bone height due to maxillary sinus pneumatization. (B) Incision line. (C and D) Lateral window approach. (E) Three implants inserted after sinus lift. (F) PRF membranes placed over sinus membrane. (G) Sticky bone. (H) Collagene membrane. (I) Flap repositioned and sutured. (J) OPG immediately after implant placement. (K) Three screw-retained solo prosthetic crowns. (L) Intraoral view.

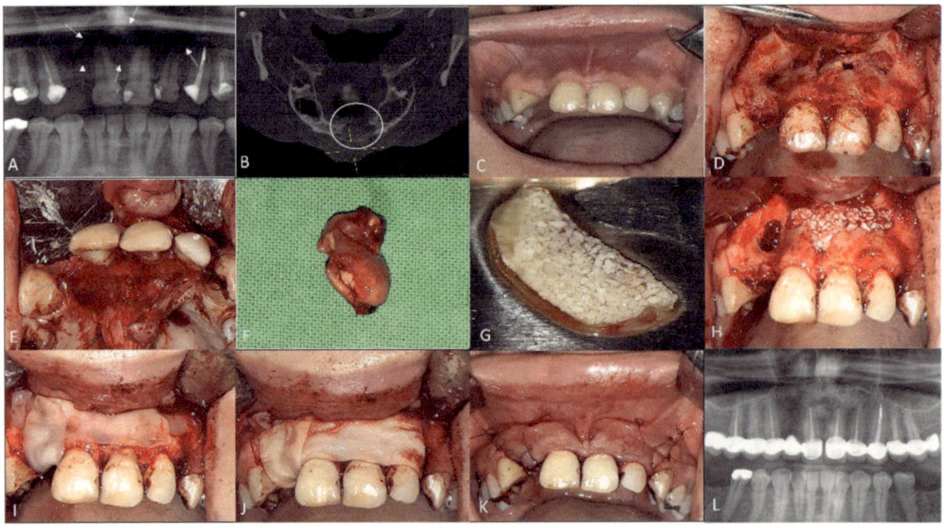

Figure 14.
Apicoectomy with large cystectomy in the maxilla. (A) Arrows pointing to large radiolucency in the maxilla. (B) Large radiolucency on CBCT image- axial view. (C) Clinical appearance. (D) Cyst destroyed vestibular cortical lamella. (E) Palatal flap raised. (F) Enucleated cyst. (G) Sticky bone. (H) Bone cavity filled with sticky bone. (I) PRF membranes. (J) Collagene membranes. (K) Flap repositioned and sutured. (L) OPG 3 months after the surgery.

5.6 Apicoectomy with extraoral fistula excision on the face

This is a very interesting case of a patient with an extraoral fistula on the face that has dental etiology (**Figure 15**). The patient had been mistreated for a longer period as the facial pathology had been considered a dermatologic condition.

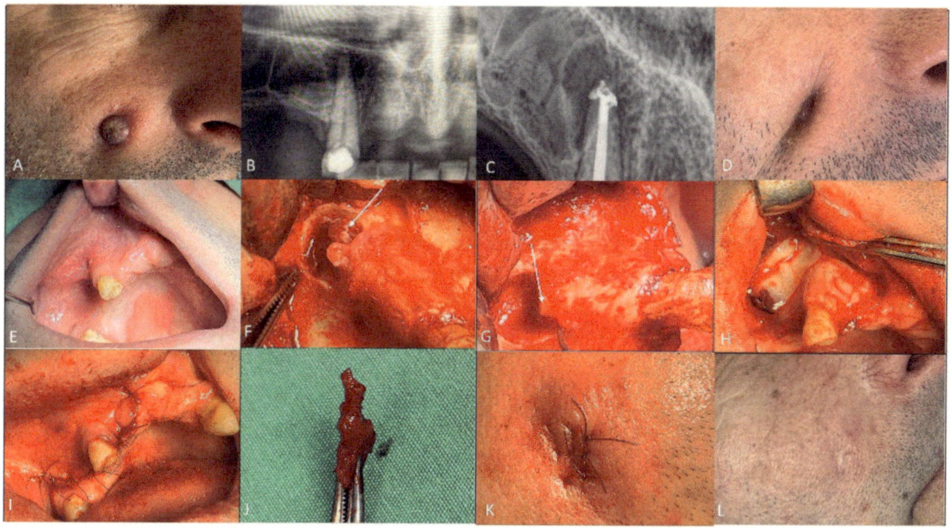

Figure 15.
Large extraoral fistula of dental origin. (A) Extraoral fistula. (B) Tooth 13 with periapical radiolucency causes the infection. (C) Definitive canal obturation. (D) The appearance of fistula during endodontic treatment. (E) Intraoral view. (F) Periapical lesion. (G) Root resected. (H) PRF membranes placed over the operating wound. (I) Flap repositioned and sutured. (J) Sinus tract. (K) Extraoral fistula was extirparted, two PRF membranes were placed in the hole, and the wound was sutured. (L) Almost invisible scar on the face.

The examination by the oral surgeon set the correct diagnosis. It was an infection of a dental etiology of tooth 13 that resulted in a periapical lesion, which was not treated and has consequently resulted in an extraoral fistula. The therapeutic approach entailed endodontic treatment of the tooth 13. During the treatment, the extraoral fistula on the face was regressing. Upon competition of definite root obturation of the tooth 13, apicoectomy ensued and was followed by the removal of the periapical bony lesion as well as excision of the canal of the fistula. For the oral wound to heal well, two PRF membranes were placed. Throughout the opening on the face, additional two PRF membranes were extraorally placed. Three months after the surgery, it can be noted (**Figure 13L**) that intraoral healing was excellent with almost unnoticeable scar extraorally.

6. Conclusion

Platelet concentrates were discovered by manipulating normal physiological processes such as hemostasis. All known platelet concentrates are high in growth factors and so have tremendous potential in regeneration processes. PRF, BIO-PRF, Alb-PRF, and sticky bone are newer generations of platelet concentrates that will influence the direction of regenerative dentistry. In the future, we may expect a greater number of clinical trials that will investigate the full potential of novel platelet concentrates.

Conflict of interest

The author declares no conflict of interest.

Notes/thanks/other declarations

I would like to thank my parents, Prof. dr Halid Sulejmanagic and Prim. dr Ajsa Ismailovic Sulejmanagic, as well as the Private Dental Clinic "Sulejmanagic," for their support during my professional and scientific development.

I'd like to thank my friend and colleague Armin Klancevic DMD for drawing **Figures 1** and **2** for this chapter.

I would like to express my gratitude to Richard Miron DDS, MSc, PhD, Dr. med. dent for donating BIO-PRF equipment to the Faculty of Dental Medicine with Clinics University of Sarajevo Bosnia and Herzegovina, which enabled me to gain new experiences in the field of novel platelet concentrates such as ALB-PRF.

Author details

Naida Hadziabdic
Faculty of Dental Medicine with Clinics, University of Sarajevo, Bosnia and Herzegovina

*Address all correspondence to: nsulejma@yahoo.com

References

[1] Costello BJ, Shah G, Kumta P, Sfeir CS. Regenerative medicine for craniomaxillofacial surgery. Oral and Maxillofacial Surgery Clinics of North America. 2010;**22**:33-42. DOI: 10.1016/j.coms.2009.10.009

[2] Miron RJ, Zucchelli G, Pikos MA, Salama M, Lee S, Guillemette V, et al. Use of platelet-rich fibrin in regenerative dentistry: A systematic review. Clinical Oral Investigations. 2017;**21**:1913-1927. DOI: 10.1007/s00784-017-2133-z

[3] Dean L. Blood and the cells it contains. National Center for Biotechnology Information (NCBI). National Library of Medicine. Bethesda, USA: National Institutes of Health; 2005

[4] Holinstat M. Normal platelet function. Cancer Metastasis Reviews. 2017;**36**:195-198. DOI: 10.1007/s10555-017-9677-x

[5] Blair P, Flaumenhaft R. Platelet α-granules: Basic biology and clinical correlates. Blood Reviews. 2009;**23**:177-189. DOI: 10.1016/j.blre.2009.04.001

[6] Prakash S, Thakur A. Platelet concentrates: Past, present and future. Journal of Maxillofacatory Oral Surgery. 2011;**10**:45-49. DOI: 10.1007/s12663-011-0182-4

[7] Coppinger J, Maguire P. Insights into the platelet releasate. Current Pharmaceutical Design. 2007;**13**:2640-2646. DOI: 10.2174/138161207781662885

[8] Chou TM, Chang HP, Wang JC. Autologous platelet concentrates in maxillofacial regenerative therapy. The Kaohsiung Journal of Medical Sciences. 2020;**36**:305-310. DOI: 10.1002/kjm2.12192

[9] Caruana A, Savina D, Macedo JP, Soares SC. From platelet-rich plasma to advanced platelet-rich fibrin: Biological achievements and clinical advances in modern surgery. European Journal of Dental. 2019;**13**:280-286. DOI: 10.1055/s-0039-1696585

[10] Dohan Ehrenfest D, Bielecki T, Mishra A, Borzini P, Inchingolo F, Sammartino G, et al. In search of a consensus terminology in the field of platelet concentrates for surgical use: Platelet-rich plasma (PRP), platelet-rich fibrin (PRF), fibrin gel polymerization and leukocytes. Current Pharmaceutical Biotechnology. 2012;**13**:1131-1137. DOI: 10.2174/138920112800624328

[11] Farina R, Bressan E, Taut A, Cucchi A, Trombelli L. Plasma rich in growth factors in human extraction sockets: A radiographic and histomorphometric study on early bone deposition. Clinical Oral Implants Research. 2013;**24**:1360-1368. DOI: 10.1111/clr.12033

[12] Dragonas P, Katsaros T, Avila-Ortiz G, Chambrone L, Schiavo JH, Palaiologou A. Effects of leukocyte–platelet-rich fibrin (L-PRF) in different intraoral bone grafting procedures: A systematic review. International Journal of Oral and Maxillofacial Surgery. 2019;**48**:250-262. DOI: 10.1016/j.ijom.2018.06.003

[13] Pavlovic V, Ciric M, Jovanovic V, Trandafilovic MS. Platelet-rich fibrin: Basics of biological actions and protocol modifications. Open Medicine. 2021;**16**:446-454

[14] Titirinli K, Tekin U, Atıl F, Önder ME, Şenguven B, Ozgul O, et al. Evaluation of advanced platelet rich

fibrin (A-PRF) on bone healing. Is it better than old version? A histological animal study. Journal of Biomaterial Tissue Engineering. 2017;7:478-483. DOI: 10.1166/jbt.2017.1592

[15] Zumarán CC, Parra MV, Olate SA, Fernández EG, Muñoz FT, Haidar ZS. The 3 R's for platelet-rich fibrin: A "super" tri-dimensional biomaterial for contemporary naturally-guided oro-maxillo-facial soft and hard tissue repair, reconstruction and regeneration. Materials (Basel). 2018;**2018**:11. DOI: 10.3390/ma11081293

[16] Pitzurra L, Jansen IDC, de Vries TJ, Hoogenkamp MA, Loos BG. Effects of L-PRF and A-PRF+ on periodontal fibroblasts in in vitro wound healing experiments. Journal of Periodontal Research. 2020;**55**:287-295. DOI: 10.1111/jre.12714

[17] El Bagdadi K, Kubesch A, Yu X, Al-Maawi S, Orlowska A, Dias A, et al. Reduction of relative centrifugal forces increases growth factor release within solid platelet-rich-fibrin (PRF)-based matrices: A proof of concept of LSCC (low speed centrifugation concept). European Journal of Trauma and Emergency Surgery. 2019;**45**:467-479. DOI: 10.1007/s00068-017-0785-7

[18] Zhang T, Dai J, Xu Y, Yu L, Wang X. Liquid phase concentrated growth factor improves autologous fat graft survival In vivo in nude mice. Aesthetic Plastic Surgery. 2021;**45**: 2417-2422. DOI: 10.1007/s00266-021-02336-x

[19] Rodella LF, Favero G, Boninsegna R, Buffoli B, Labanca M, Scarì G, et al. Growth factors, CD34 positive cells, and fibrin network analysis in concentrated growth factors fraction. Microscopy Research and Technique. 2011;**74**:772-777. DOI: 10.1002/jemt.20968

[20] de Barros Mourão A, Gheno E, Lourenço E, Barbosa RL, Kurtzman G, Javid K, et al. Characterization of a new membrane from concentrated growth factors associated with denaturized albumin (Alb-CGF) for clinical applications: A preliminary study. International Journal of Growth Factors Stem Cells. 2018;**1**:64. DOI: 10.4103/gfsc.gfsc_21_18

[21] Miron RJ, Chai J, Zheng S, Feng M, Sculean A, Zhang Y. A novel method for evaluating and quantifying cell types in platelet rich fibrin and an introduction to horizontal centrifugation. Journal Biomedical Material Research—Part A. 2019;**107**:2257-2271. DOI: 10.1002/jbm.a.36734

[22] Miron RJ, Chai J, Zhang P, Li Y, Wang Y, et al. A novel method for harvesting concentrated platelet-rich fibrin (C-PRF) with a 10-fold increase in platelet and leukocyte yields. Clinical Oral Investigations. 2020;**24**:2819-2828. DOI: 10.1007/s00784-019-03147-w

[23] Kawase T, Kamiya M, Kobayashi M, Tanaka T, Okuda K, Wolff LF, et al. The heat-compression technique for the conversion of platelet-rich fibrin preparation to a barrier membrane with a reduced rate of biodegradation. Journal of Biomedical Material Research. 2015;**103**:825-831. DOI: 10.1002/jbm.b.33262

[24] Fujioka-Kobayashi M, Schaller B, Mourão CFDAB, Zhang Y, Sculean A, Miron RJ. Biological characterization of an injectable platelet-rich fibrin mixture consisting of autologous albumin gel and liquid platelet-rich fibrin (Alb-PRF). Platelets. 2021;**32**:74-81. DOI: 10.1080/09537104.2020.1717455

[25] Upadhayaya V, Arora A, Goyal A. Bioactive platelet aggregates: Prp, Prgf, Prf, Cgf and sticky bone. IOSR Journal of

Dental Medical Science. 2017;**16**:05-11. DOI: 10.9790/0853-1605060511

[26] Khadher A. Ethoss versus mineralized plasmatic matrix for maxillary lateral sinus lifting with simultaneous implant placement. Mansoura Journal of Dental. 2022;**9**:38-44. DOI: 10.21608/mjd.2022.241150

[27] Abdelfadil E, Aboelmaaty W. Mineralized plasmatic matrix for horizontal ridge augmentation in anterior maxilla with and without a covering collagen membrane. The Open Dentistry Journal. 2021;**14**:743-751. DOI: 10.2174/1874210602014010743

[28] Samir E, Hicham S, Keltoum EO, Zouheir I. Management of post-extractional alveolar socket with mineralized plasmatic matrix before implant placement: A case report. Asian Pacific Journal of Health Science. 2017;**4**:220-227. DOI: 10.21276/apjhs.2017.4.3.33

[29] Sghaireen M, Ganji K, Alam M, Rahman S, Billah S. Mineralized plasmatic matrix in ridge preservation: A randomized controlled clinical trial. The International Journal of Periodontics & Restorative Dentistry. 2021;**41**:e103-e112. DOI: 10.11607/prd.4972

[30] Sghaireen MG, Alzarea BK, Alam MK, Rahman SA, Ganji KK, Alhabib S, et al. Implant stability, bone graft loss and density with conventional and mineralized plasmatic matrix bone graft preparations-a randomized crossover trial. Journal of Hard Tissue Biology. 2020;**29**:273-278. DOI: 10.2485/jhtb.29.273

[31] Al-fakhrany AH, Shuman MA, Tawfik BA. Evaluation of mineralized plasmatic matrix graft after surgical removal of impacted mandibular third molars (Randomized clinical study). Al-Azhar Journal of Dental Science. 2017;**20**:53-63. DOI: 10.21608/ajdsm.2017.107490

[32] Mansour A, Khalil M, Shuman M. Evaluation of mineralized plasmatic matrix as a grafting material around immediate dental implant in mandibular posterior teeth. Al-Azhar Journal of Dental Science. 2021;**24**:297-305. DOI: 10.21608/ajdsm.2020.38219.1088

[33] Eldidi LM, Abdelhamid AM, Hommos AM, Eldakkak SM, El Zawawy HT. Evaluation of using mineralized plasmatic matrix in osseous regeneration. Alexandria Dental Journal. 2019;**44**:81-86. DOI: 10.21608/adjalexu.2019.57583

[34] Amine K, Gharibi A, Hsaine A, Kissa J. Effect of bone regeneration with mineralized plasmatic matrix for implant placement in aesthetic zone. Case Report Dental. 2017;**2017**:10-15. DOI: 10.1155/2017/2639564

[35] Mohamed MS, Sc M, Elsharkawy AT, Abd- AH. Evaluation of mineralized plasmatic matrix prepared from allogenic bone graft in alveolar cleft closure: A prospective randomized. Triple Blinded, Parallel Clinical Trial. 2021;**25**:14669-14685

[36] El Moheb M, Al-Zarea B, Sghaireen MG, Toriya J, Mizohata A, Patil S, et al. Mineralized plasmatic matrix to enhance the bone grafting technique. Journal of Hard Tissue Biology. 2017;**26**:289-292. DOI: 10.2485/jhtb.26.289

[37] Nadon F, Chaput B, Perisse J, De Berail A, Lauwers F, Lopez R. Interest of mineralized plasmatic matrix in secondary autogenous bone graft for the treatment of alveolar clefts. The Journal of Craniofacial Surgery. 2015;**26**:2148-2151. DOI: 10.1097/SCS.0000000000001951

[38] Ellapakurthi P, Reddy GSP. The effectiveness of mineralized plasmatic matrix in the closure of alveolar clefts with volumetric assessment. Regeneration Medical Research. 2021;**9**:1. DOI: 10.1051/rmr/210004

[39] Chandra R, Shivateja K, Reddy A. Autogenous bone ring transplant vs autologous growth factor–enriched bone graft matrix in extraction sockets with deficient buccal bone: A comparative clinical study. The International Journal of Oral & Maxillofacial Implants. 2019;**34**:1424-1433. DOI: 10.11607/jomi.7614

[40] Chehata I, Monim G, Refahee S. Effect of mineralized plasmatic matrix. Egyptian Dental Journal. 2020;**66**:2153-2164

[41] Ghanaati S, Mourão C, Adam E, Sader R, Zadeh H, Al-Maawi S. The role of centrifugation process in the preparation of therapeutic blood concentrates: Standardization of the protocols to improve reproducibility. International Journal of Growth Factors Stem Cells Dental. 2019;**2**:41. DOI: 10.4103/gfsc.gfsc_15_19

[42] Miron RJ, Pinto NR, Quirynen M, Ghanaati S. Standardization of relative centrifugal forces in studies related to platelet-rich fibrin. Journal of Periodontology. 2019;**90**:817-820. DOI: 10.1002/JPER.18-0553

[43] Margolis J. Glass surface and blood coagulation. Nature. 1956;**178**:805-806. DOI: 10.1038/178805b0

[44] Miron RJ, Kawase T, Dham A, Zhang Y, Fujioka-Kobayashi M, Sculean A. A technical note on contamination from PRF tubes containing silica and silicone. BMC Oral Health. 2021;**21**:1-11. DOI: 10.1186/s12903-021-01497-0

[45] Masuki H, Isobe K, Kawabata H, Tsujino T, Yamaguchi S, Watanabe T, et al. Acute cytotoxic effects of silica microparticles used for coating of plastic blood-collection tubes on human periosteal cells. Odontology. 2020;**108**:545-552. DOI: 10.1007/s10266-020-00486-z

[46] Tsujino T, Masuki H, Nakamura M, Isobe K. Striking differences in platelet distribution between advanced-platelet-rich fibrin and concentrated growth factors: Effects of silica-containing plastic tubes. Journal of Functional Biomaterials. 2019;**10**:43. DOI: 10.3390/jfb10030043

[47] Miron RJ, Horrocks NA, Zhang Y, Horrocks G, Pikos MA, Sculean A. Extending the working properties of liquid platelet-rich fibrin using chemically modified PET tubes and the bio-cool device. Clinical Oral Investigations. 2022;**26**:2873-2878. DOI: 10.1007/s00784-021-04268-x

Chapter 5

A Review of Current Surgical Approaches and Diagnostic Features Associated with Craniosynostosis Patients and the Relation to Oral and Maxillofacial Surgery

Robert Pellecchia, Kambiz Vatandoost, Anirudh Nair, Farajollah Soleimanzadeh, Benjamin Richardson and Gunanand D. Persaud III

Abstract

The chapter will describe etiology of craniosynostosis and the management in the young child. Included will be classification of various forms of craniosynostosis and surgical management. Diagnostic imaging including CT scan, MRI, etc. will be mentioned as a tool in the treatment considerations of the patient with Craniosynostosis. Initial diagnosis, and consultation with appropriate surgical service, and treatment options will be discussed in the Chapter. Surgical options will include surgical plan and fixation methods. Further discussion of combined orthodontic and surgical treatment planning is presented. Complications will be discussed and summarized including reasonable expectations with both short and long term outcomes.

Keywords: sutures, syndromic, craniosynostosis, oral surgery, maxillofacial surgery

1. Introduction

Craniosynostosis is a "developmental craniofacial anomaly, resulting in impairment of brain development and abnormally shaped skull" [1]. It involves premature fusion of the sutures of cranial vault in-utero. If untreated, over time craniosynostosis can cause significant cognitive and neurological impairments. Various diagnostic, surgical, and post-operative considerations should be appreciated in order to avoid unnecessary long-term systemic issues in patients with this condition.

This disorder can be classified into three different categories depending upon its formation:

- "If a craniosynostosis develops due to a primary defect of the ossification process it is called primary craniosynostosis" [1].
- Secondary craniosynostosis develops as a "result of known systemic diseases with hematologic or metabolic dysfunction" [1].
- It can also be divided into either syndromic or non-syndromic craniosynostosis which involves the development of this disorder as a result of another existing condition such as Pfeiffer syndrome or an isolated disorder, respectively. Syndromic craniosynostosis accounts for approximately 40% of reported cases and tends to have a genetic involvement (**Table 1**). Furthermore, this disorder can also be classified as either simple or complex where "simple craniosynostosis is a term used when only one suture fuses prematurely, while complex craniosynostosis is used to describe a premature fusion of multiple sutures" [1].

Certain conditions can increase the risk at which a child can develop craniosynostosis such as "family history of abnormal head shapes, in utero exposure to teratogenic drugs, intrauterine restrains, or an abnormal fetal position, as well as any complications during pregnancy and any delayed milestones" [1]. As a result of this, it is essential to perform a thorough examination on the medical history of the patient.

Typically, craniosynostosis is a disorder that is diagnosable within the first year of life. Diagnosis is performed by a "clinical assessment that checks for its presence, whether or not the development of this disorder is a result of an associated syndrome, and if elective or urgent management is required" [1]. Common characteristics of the various classifications of craniosynostosis are summarized in **Table 2**. If surgical treatment is to be taken, then the diagnosis will be confirmed radiologically, either by computed tomography (CT), radiography, or magnetic resonance imaging (MRI). Radiography is the most common method used to confirm the presence of craniosynostosis as it is cost effective, does not require the use of anesthesia, and mitigates the risk of radiation exposure. One exception to the use of radiology to confirm the presence of craniosynostosis is when this disorder is classified as syndromic craniosynostosis. Genetic testing is used for "patients presenting coronal or multi-suture synostosis, since these two types are often genetically determined" [1].

Genes Involved in Syndromic Craniosynostosis	
Clinical diagnosis	**Genes to be investigated**
Apert	*FGFR2*
Crouzon	*FGFR2*
Crouzon with acanthosis nigricans	*FGFR3*
Pfeiffer	*FGFR2* (*FGFR1*)
Carpenter	*RAB23*
Muenke	*FGFR3* (*TWIST1*)
Saethre-Chotzen	*TWIST1* (*FGFR3*)
Craniofrontonasal dysplasia	*EFNB1*

Table 1.
Gene involvements in syndromic craniosynostosis [2].

Type of craniosynostosis	Typical characteristics
Scaphocephaly	• Premature fusion of the sagittal suture • Elongated head in the anterior-posterior and shortened in the bilateral direction • Frontal bossing is present • Boys more frequently affected (3.5:1) • Premature fusion of the coronal suture • Forehead flattened on the affected side • High supraorbital margins (Harlequin sign)
Anterior plagiocephaly	• Forehead pushed forward on the unaffected side • Nasal septum deviation towards the normal side • More common in girls (2:1) • Unilateral lambdoid synostosis
Posterior plagiocephaly	• Frontal and occipital bossing • Ipsilateral ear and mastoid displaced downward • Head shape from above may resemble a trapezoid • Ipsilateral ear and forehead displaced anteriorly • Parallelogram shape of the head
Positional plagiocephaly	• Ipsilateral occipital flattening accompanied by contralateral occipital bossing • Male to female ratio 3:1 • Premature fusion of the metopic suture
Trigonocephaly	• Occipital part is broad, forehead is narrow and pointed • Triangular shape of the head • Hypotelorism • Bilateral coronal synostosis • Short skull • Forehead and occipital part flattened
Brachycephaly	• Frontal bone prominent and elongated in vertical direction • Hypertelorism • Harlequin malformation of the orbits

Table 2.
Common characteristics of types of craniosynostosis [1].

Once the type of craniosynostosis is identified, there are two treatment options available:

One option is to perform an endoscopic suturectomy which is only performed on "patients less than six months of age because the bone is more flexible and manageable by an endoscope. The postoperative recovery is faster, there is less blood loss, and the surgery is shorter compared to open craniotomy. The only downside is that most times, there is a need to combine the surgery with the postoperative use of a remodeling helmet for 4 to 6 months" [3].

A second option that involves surgery is an open craniotomy. This procedure is performed on "patients older than six months because the bones are more rigid and cannot be manipulated as well with an endoscope. This modality allows for a better

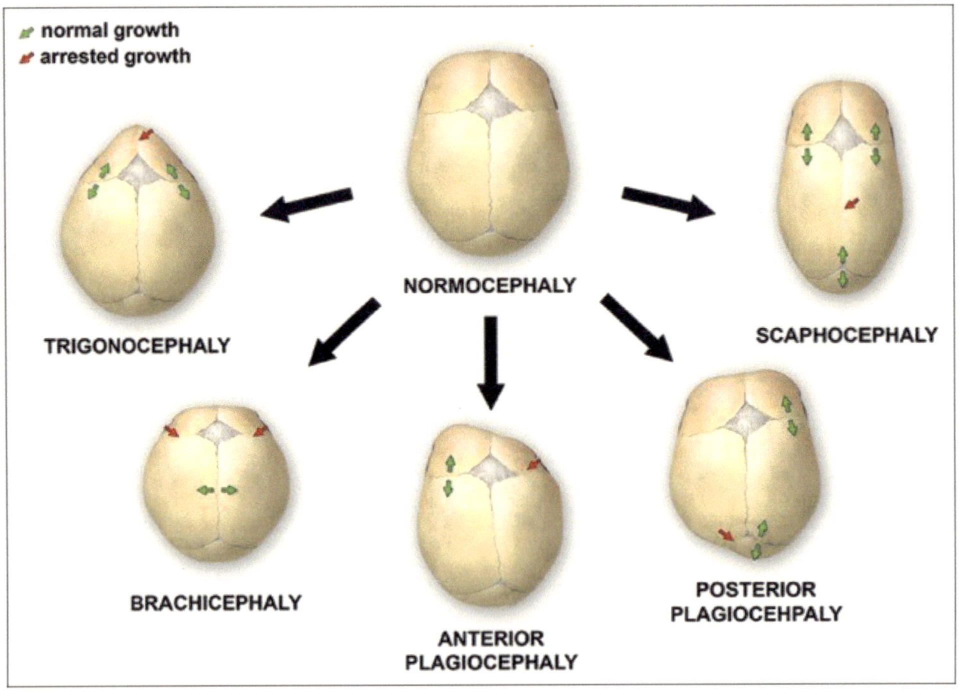

Figure 1.
Visual depictions of the various types of simple synostoses (Kadjic et al).

remodeling of the skull and decreases the need for helmet use postoperatively" [3]. Ideally, surgery should be done "between 6 and 12 months of age when there are no signs of increased ICP or airway compromise" [3].

The objective that open craniotomies and endoscopic suturectomies aim to accomplish is to "create enough space in the cranial vault for the brain to grow and develop properly as well as to provide the child with a more decent-looking appearance" [3]. While these procedures tend to be conclusive in their ability to resolve this disorder, continuous treatment and follow-ups are often required in cases where the patient has syndromic craniosynostosis (**Figure 1**).

1.1 Scaphocephaly

This type of synostosis occurs due to a premature fusion of the sagittal suture and is more commonly found in premature infants. It can be detected due to the elongation of the head in the anterior-posterior direction along with the shortening of the head in the bilateral direction. Another observable indicator of the presence of scaphocephaly is the possibility of frontal bossing along with a noticeable ridge along the sagittal suture. "Boys are more frequently affected than girls, with a ratio of 3.5:1" [1].

1.2 Anterior Plagiocephaly

Anterior plagiocephaly occurs when the coronal suture fuses prematurely. Observable signs of this type of synostosis involve a flattening of the forehead on the affected side, a protruding forehead on the unaffected side, and a nasal septum deviation towards the normal side. If a radiograph is performed, anyone that has anterior plagiocephaly will display a characteristic reading that is more commonly known as a Harlequin sign due to the high supraorbital margins that the affected have. In some cases where the "bicoronal fusion" closes prematurely, the condition is called brachycephaly" [1]. This type of synostosis affects girls more than boys in a 2:1 ratio.

1.3 Posterior Plagiocephaly

"Posterior plagiocephaly is a unilateral lambdoid synostosis" [1]. Distinguishable signs to look out for include frontal or occipital bossing, a displacement of the ipsilateral ear and mastoid downwards, and depending on the severity of the posterior plagiocephaly, the head may look like a trapezoid when viewed from above.

1.4 Trigonocephaly

"Trigonocephaly results from a premature fusion of the metopic suture" [1]. Prominent features that are unique to the presence of trigonocephaly are a broad back of the head, a pointed forehead that appears to be triangular when viewed from above. The orbits are also closer together than normal which is commonly referred to as hypotelorism. The ratio of boys to girls affected by this type of synostosis is 3.3:1.

1.5 Brachycephaly

"Brachycephaly is a bilateral coronal synostosis" [1]. It is common for those affected by brachycephaly to display signs such as a flattened forehead or occipital bone along with a "frontal bone [that] is prominent and elongated in a vertical direction" [1]. The orbits are also further apart than normal which is commonly referred to as hypertelorism. This separation can be picked up on radiographs. Studies also tend to show that brachycephaly is typically a type of synostosis that is heavily influenced by genetics or develops as a result of syndromic craniosynostosis.

Characteristic	Non-synostotic (deformational) plagiocephaly	Synostotic plagiocephaly
Cause/definition	Abnormally shaped head due to external forces applied to the skull, not due to craniosynostosis	Premature fusion of one or more cranial sutures; exact cause unknown; genetic and environmental factors may play a role
Common types	Lateral deformational (positional) plagiocephaly; posterior deformational plagiocephaly (positional brachycephaly)	Bilateral coronal craniosynostosis (synostotic brachycephaly); sagittal cranosynostosis (dolichocephaly/>scaphocephaly); metopic craniosynostosis (trogonocepnaly)
Distinguishing features	Round, symmetrical head shape at birth; parallelogram or brachycephalic head shape: ear may be anteriorly displaced; no palpable bony ridges	May have abnormal head shape at birth; trapezoid head shape; ear may be posteriorly displaced; palpable bony ridges
Management	Repositioning and physical therapy; helmet in some cases	Usually surgery; helmet in some cases

Note: Adapted from **Tables 1** *and* **2** *in Nield et al., 2007.*

Table 3.
Comparison of non-synostotic (deformational) plagiocephaly and synostotic plagiocephaly [4, 5].

1.6 Deformational Plagiocephaly

Deformation or non-synostotic plagiocephaly is unlike any other type of plagiocephaly as it is not synostotic. **Table 3** summarizes the key differences between non-synostotic and synostotic plagiocephaly. It develops as a result of continuous pressure to one area of the head. It is hard to distinguish between the two as some of the physical changes that come about as a result of deformational plagiocephaly can be similar to those found in synostotic plagiocephaly. However, the physical changes that arise as a result of deformational plagiocephaly can be resolved with time and by changing the sides that the baby sleeps on whereas synostotic plagiocephaly requires surgery to remedy any physical changes. Due to the number of babies that sleep in a supine position in order to avoid the risk of cot death, the amount of deformational plagiocephaly cases rose from "20% to 48% since the early 1990's" [2, 6] which makes it harder to detect cases in which craniosynostosis is present.

2. Approaches to the management of craniosynostosis

There are various approaches a surgeon should consider for treatment planning a patient with craniosynostosis.

2.1 Surgical approaches

Most occurrences require timely surgical correction. Various articles highlight the importance of the patient's age as the predominant factor when determining the surgical approach. Per Chong et al.: for patients younger than 6 months, a minimally invasive procedure should be considered. This most commonly involves a minimally invasive suturectomy with postoperative helmet therapy.

The goal of minimally invasive suturectomy is to release a fused suture with small exposure. Chong et al. outlines their approach to a case of sagittal craniosynostosis:

> *"The patient is prepared with the head extended in a prone position. Skin preparation is done with povidone-iodine. Two transverse incisions are made of 3–4 cm length at 1 cm behind the anterior fontanelle and 1 cm in front of the lambdoid suture. An additional incision may be needed between the two sites to manipulate safely in a patient with a longer head. A subperiosteal dissection is made along the desired craniectomy site. Burr holes are placed over the fused suture at both incision sites. The dura is dissected and carefully detached from the fused bone. During these procedures, a fiber optic suction tip or endoscope is used for the safe and accurate manipulation of the compromising space. Strip craniectomy is performed using curved Mayo scissors, sternal scissors and straight rongeurs. The fused bone is removed from the anterior fontanelle anteriorly to the lambda posteriorly. The width of the craniectomy site is targeted to be between 3 cm to 4 cm. After the strip craniectomy, additional lateral wedge osteotomies or barrel stave osteotomies might be conducted according to the surgeon's preference. Bleeding from the diploic space is controlled by bone wax and monopolar electrocautery. With the insertion of a drain, the wound is closed layer by layer" [7].*

Postoperative helmet therapy is typically initiated after subgaleal swelling is reduced and all stitches are removed. The helmet is recommended to be worn for

12–18 months to account for this important rapid brain and skull growth period. One helmet may be sufficient depending on the procedure (such as following sagittal craniosynostosis) or the patient may require two or more helmet adjustments. An orthotist fits patients for the helmet.

2.1.1 Fronto-orbital advancement

The goal of the fronto-orbital advancement (FOA) surgical technique is to create space in the skull while reshaping the forehead and the orbit. FOA is indicated in unicoronal, bicoronal, or metopic craniosynostosis.

In this procedure, a coronal incision is performed using a sinusoidal pattern with hemostatic clips. Subperiosteal dissection is performed to raise the anterior scalp flap to expose the superior orbital rim and orbital roof bilaterally. Caution must be taken with the release of the supraorbital neurovascular bundle from its notch and retraction with gentle pressure on the globe. The subperiosteal dissection is then directed laterally to expose the fronto-zygomatic suture and lateral orbital wall and medially to expose the nasal root and medial orbital walls. The lateral canthus is released while the medial canthus must remain intact. A frontal craniotomy is performed, diligently avoiding the patent sutures, and frontal bone flap is removed with care to avoid damage to the sagittal sinus and the dura. Any bleeding from inadvertent damage to the dura must be controlled immediately after removal of the frontal bone. Superior osteotomy from anterior to posterior is created, followed by the lateral osteotomy through the zygomatic-frontal suture [8].

Intracranially, an osteotomy of the orbital roof is performed through the anterior cranial fossa while protecting the frontal lobe and globe, as well as the temporal lobe when extending laterally to the lateral sphenoid. A nasal frontal osteotomy is performed starting laterally and extending it medially to avoid damage to the dura. Once the osteotomies are released, the bones, except for the frontal bone, are gently bent to the desired contour, rearranged with overcorrection to avoid relapse. The frontal bone flap is transected, molded and reattached with absorbable hardware and/or sutures in an overcorrected anterior to posterior position to avoid relapse. The sites are irrigated with copious amounts of saline and closed in a layered fashion (**Figure 2**) [8].

2.1.2 Posterior cranial vault distraction

The posterior cranial vault distraction (PCVD) technique has been used with the goal of increasing intracranial volume while achieving desired cosmetic results. With low perioperative complications, this procedure allows for 25–30% increase in intracranial volume. Salokorpi et al. describes their method of PCVD with virtual surgical planning preoperatively for osteotomy lines, size of bone flap, direction of distraction and location of the distraction devices.

A coronal incision is performed in a weave fashion and the location of the incision should be placed to allow for front-orbital expansion procedure, if needed. The dissection in the occipital area is performed subperiosteally. Once marked, the osteotomy is performed using the preoperative plan. Burr holes are made with a ball drill with caution to avoid dural damage. The burr holes are also placed, bilaterally, on the lambdoid sutures. The dura is dissected through the burr holes and further craniotomy is performed starting from the temporal and extending to the sagittal suture. The craniotomy is then extended occipitally over the posterior sinus structures. Bleeding in the occipital area from the emissary veins must be managed with

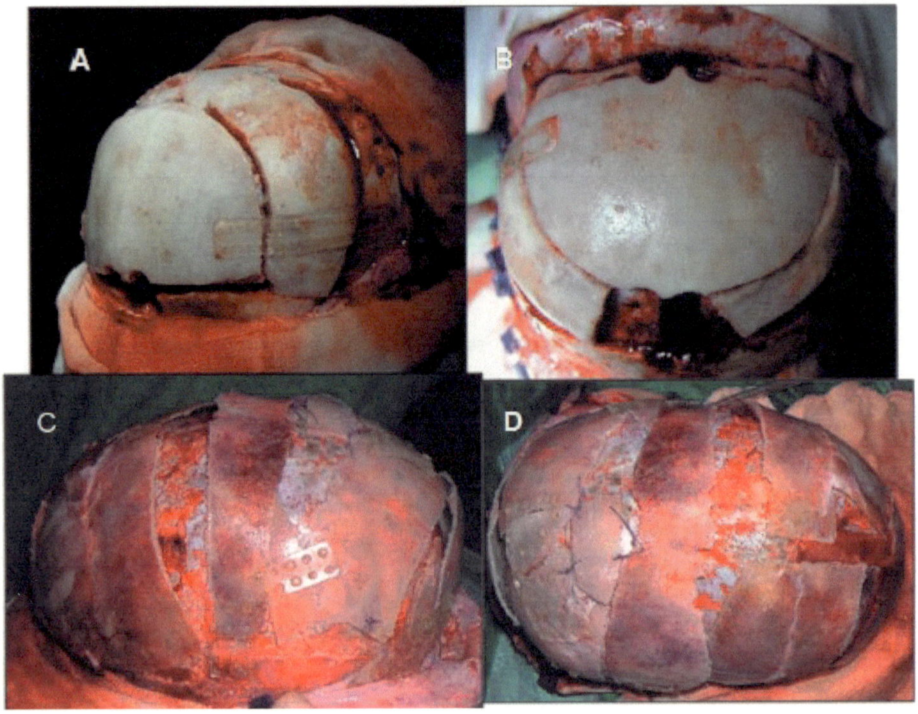

Figure 2.
Bilateral fronto-orbtal advancement [A, B]. Total vault remodeling [C, D] [9, 10].

bone wax and hemostatic matrix with thrombin. A short bone bridge is left to ensure stability during fixation of the distractors. After fixation, this bone bridge is cut [11].

Distractors are placed, parallel to each other, in the locations that were planned preoperatively. Salokorpi et al. preferred to position the devices with anterior positioning of the activation arms. The occipital movement of the flap is confirmed by activating the devices for a few millimeters. The bone is left attached to the dura as detachment increases the risk of bleeding from venous sinuses. Salokorpi reports that a full mobilization of the bone flap does not affect the ossification. Postoperatively, after a latency period of 5–7 days, the rate of distraction is performed at 0.5–1 mm/day in one to two sessions per day. Once sufficient ossification is obtained, the devices can be removed with small skin cuts perpendicular to the coronal incision [11].

2.1.3 Endoscopic strip craniectomy

The goal of endoscopic strip craniectomy is to perform a strip craniectomy using an endoscope to minimize scalp incision, blood loss, operative times and postoperative recovery periods. The use of the endoscope to perform the strip craniectomy was described by Barone and Jiminez, published in Plastic and Reconstructive Surgery in 1999.

Two 2 cm incisions are placed; one of the posterior aspect of the anterior fontanelle and the other over the lambda. With the use of an endoscope, dissection is performed in the subgaleal plane between these two incisions and extending to the bitemporal regions. With endoscopic visualization, electrocautery is performed for hemostasis to create a dry subgaleal dissection. Then, blunt dissection is performed to separate the dura from the bony edge of the fontanelle. A rongeur is used to remove a thin strip of bone anterior to the lambdoid suture to avoid injury to the sagittal sinus. Dura is dissected off the lambda and posterior aspect of the sagittal suture. With direct visualization, the sagittal sinus is carefully peeled off the synostosed sagittal suture. Epidural dissection is extended laterally to the level of the squamosal suture. Once complete subgaleal and epidural exposure is obtained, a lateral paramedian osteotomy is made using bone cutting scissors and a midline strip measuring 1.5–7 cm wide and 7–12 cm long is removed. Wedges of bone are removed and the surgical field is irrigated with antibiotic solution prior to closure. Postoperatively, Barone and Jiminez describe that the patients were placed in custom-made helmets with continued molding therapy for upto 8 months [12].

Lambdoid, metopic and coronal synostosis follow similar techniques except for some modifications. In lambdoid sutures, incisions are planned preoperatively using ECG and plain x-ray film and the patient is placed in a full prone position. In metopic and coronal synostosis, the patient is placed in supine position and an incision is made at the hairline centrally. Additionally, the subgaleal dissection is performed with the endoscope to the nasofrontal suture (**Figure 3**) [12].

2.1.4 Spring-mediated cranioplasty

Spring-mediated cranioplasty is a surgical technique employed for the correction of sagittal craniosynostosis to expand the parietal bones transversely to reverse midvault disproportion.

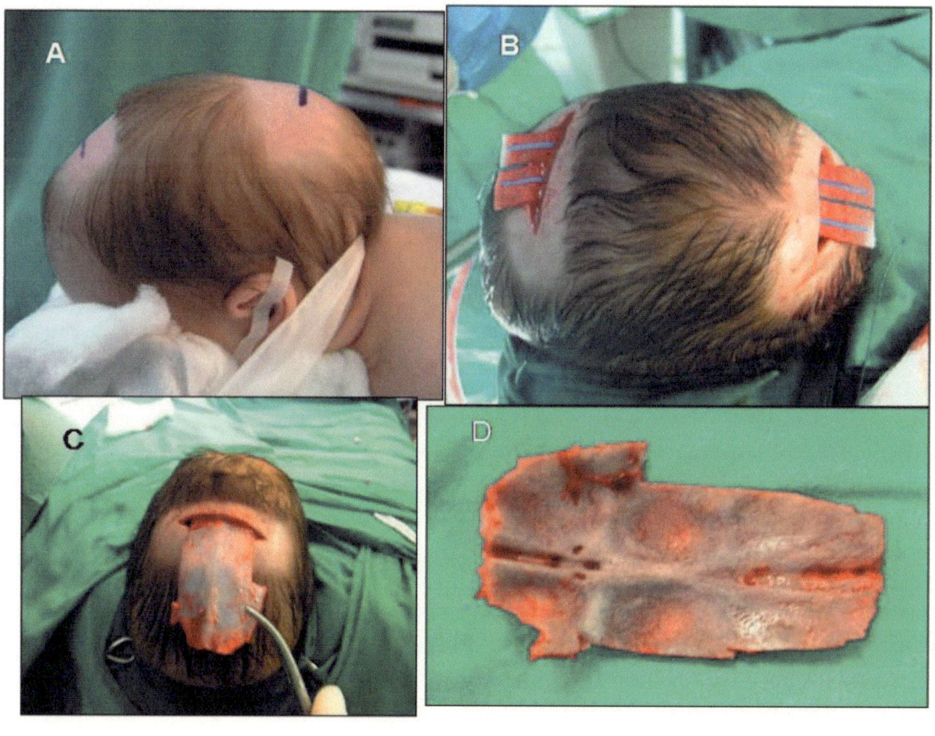

Figure 3.
Patient with scaphocephaly treated with endoscopic-assisted suturectomy and osteotomies. Patient in modified prone position [A]. Surgical patties showing subcutaneous dissection [B]. Sagittal suture excision [C]. Excised sagittal suture [D] [10].

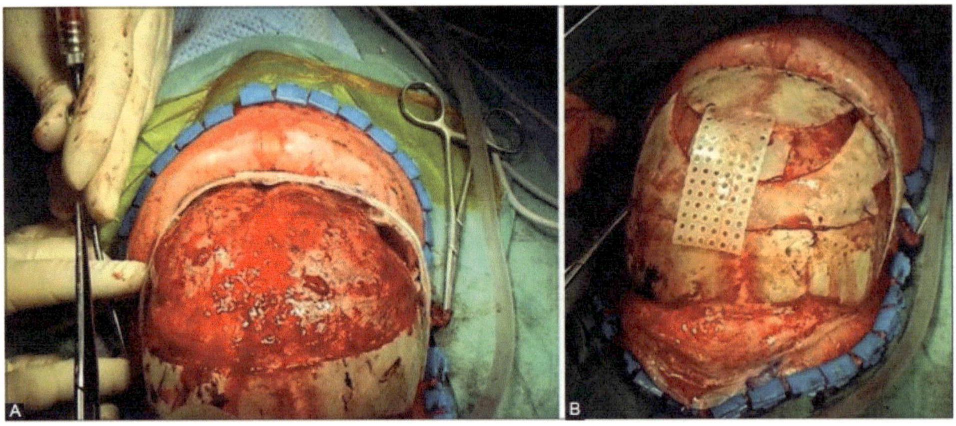

Figure 4.
Image of craniosynostosis surgery being performed on a patient with anterior plagiocephaly. Bicoronal flap exposing defect [A]. Completed skull reconstruction with resorbable plates [B] [13].

Two transverse incisions are made posterior to the anterior fontanelle and anterior to the posterior fontanelle allowing easier access to the most distal anterior and posterior aspects of the sagittal suture to perform the craniectomy and placing the distractor springs. After identifying and elevating the subgaleal plane, burr holes are placed at the midline of the inferior and superior incisions. The inferior and superior incisions depend on the prone or supine positioning of the patient. A craniectomy is performed and three strips, 1.5 cm or less in width, are removed. Following this, cranial springs, that were selected preoperatively with the criteria of length, thickness and U bend, are placed in the anterior, mid-vault and posterior positions. The springs are placed 1 cm posterior to the anterior fontanelle, 1 cm anterior to the lambdoid sutures and at the parietal bone midpoint. Following copious irrigation, the incisions are closed in a layered fashion (**Figure 4**) [14].

2.2 Combined surgical and orthodontic approach

Treatment of craniosynostosis involves a care team that includes but is not limited to an oral maxillofacial surgeon, neurosurgeon, pediatric dentist, plastic surgeon, pediatric neurologist, geneticist, plastic surgeon, dentist, and orthodontist. As a result of the various medicinal disciplines that are involved in the care of a patient that has craniosynostosis, treatments that the patients undergo are a joint effort that requires the cooperation of those involved. A common collaboration that is vital to providing care for patients afflicted by craniosynostosis is that of dentists and surgeons. While surgeons perform operations on a patient, dentists can monitor the patient and keep record of the recovery process using "photographs, diagnostic models, and imaging records" [1]. Dentists are also heavily involved in ensuring that the teeth of the patient develop properly. **Table 4** below illustrates the reliance of providers on the various types of recommended interventions to manage orthodontic patients:

Severe cases of craniosynostosis (typically syndromic craniosynostosis) often present an array of problems that need to be dealt with in a timely manner to ensure that the patient does not suffer from any mortal symptoms. While the table above outlines a general treatment plan for a patient that has craniosynostosis, those that suffer from syndromic craniosynostosis require certain steps in their treatment plan

Age (y)	Dentition Stage	Interventions	Providers involved
<1	Primary dentition	Establish dental home	Pediatric dentist
1–6	Primary dentition	• Periodic oral examinations • Assessments for growth • Supervised oral hygiene practices/aids • Maxillary expansion when possible to facilitate incisor and molar eruption	Pediatric dentist, orthodontist, and oral and maxillofacial surgeon
7–12	Mixed dentition	• Oral hygiene assessments and prophylaxis as needed • Phase I orthodontic treatment (e.g., maxillary expansion to correct posterior crossbites, limited maxillary arch orthodontic treatment to correct anterior crossbites, limited orthodontic treatment to facilitate eruption of permanent dentition, and reverse-pull headgear treatment) • Sequential extractions of primary teeth to facilitate eruption of permanent teeth • Midface advancement (as needed)	Pediatric dentist, periodontist, orthodontist, and oral and maxillofacial surgeon
13–21	Permanent dentition	• Periodic oral examinations, hygiene assessments, and prophylaxis • Comprehensive phase of orthodontic treatment with or without orthognathic surgery (depending on degree of skeletal imbalance) • Restorative treatment (eg, implants, crowns, veneers) following completion of comprehensive phase of orthodontic treatment	Orthodontist, oral and maxillofacial surgeon, periodontist, and prosthodontist
>21	Permanent dentition	• Retention checks • Periodic observations to assess long-term stability of surgical corrections • Periodic oral hygiene visits	Orthodontist, oral and maxillofacial surgeon, and periodontist

Table 4.
Outline of a treatment plan for a patient with craniosynostosis [1].

to be performed earlier or later. For example, patients with syndromic craniosynostosis tend to develop severe midface hypoplasia and suffer from “sleep apnea as a result of retropalatal airway collapse” [1]. In cases such as these, it is imperative that patients undergo premature midface advancement surgery in order to remedy the discomfort associated with sleep apnea along with fixing the patient’s facial profile. In conjunction with the midface advancement surgery, orthodontic treatment is also performed in order to ensure that the patient can attain a normal occlusion. Typically, this process involves maxillary expansion to allow for incisors and molars to have space to grow in the mouth. “Depending on the severity of maxillary arch constriction, several rounds of expansion may be required” [1]. This process is outlined by Azoulay et al. in a case where they deal with a patient that has syndromic craniosynostosis as a result of Pfeiffer syndrome.

“It is best to use a 4-banded expansion appliance if adequate anterior (primary first molars or primary canines) and posterior abutments (permanent first molars) are present, and overexpansion (by about 30%) should be achieved to account for expected relapse. The expansion appliance (usually hyrax, W arch, or quad helix) should be in place for at least 3 months and a fixed transpalatal arch with mesial extension arms should be placed at the time of device removal. Hawley appliances (with acrylic covering of the palate) can also be used, but these need to be periodically adjusted as the primary teeth exfoliate and permanent teeth emerge. It is most efficient to correct transverse maxillary deficiency during the mixed dentition phase when the circum-maxillary and palatal sutures are patent. As the patient ages, the palatal suture becomes fused and there is a considerable amount of resistance from the circum-maxillary sutures to maxillary expansion. In such situations, a surgically assisted maxillary expansion may be required" [1].

The procedure described above outlines one of the phases of orthodontic treatment that a patient with craniosynostosis goes through. In addition to this treatment there are other steps that can be divided into presurgical orthodontics, orthognathic surgery, and postsurgical orthodontics. Before undergoing maxillary/mandibular surgery to fully correct the patient's occlusion it is necessary for some pre-surgery setup to be done. The objectives of this stage are to align and level both maxillary and mandibular arches, obtain compatible arch forms, remove dental compensations, and resolve crowding/spacing issues [1]. After the patient has undergone the necessary prerequisite treatments, single jaw or bimaxillary surgery is performed "to correct anterior/posterior, transverse, and vertical maxillary/mandibular discrepancies" [1]. Finally, the patient is left with a normal occlusion that needs minor touchup and detailing which is accomplished in the postsurgery phase of orthodontics.

3. Complications

There are a wide range of surgical complications that can present following the above mentioned procedures. The primary complications can be summarized in **Table 5**.

Esparza et al. discuss the various complications they found in a review of 283 cases. Mortality was very low with only 2 of their 283 patients reported death 1 year following the procedure with the cause of death owing more to the patient's syndrome

Complications of surgery
Wound infection
Intraoperative bleeding
Postoperative hematoma (subgaleal, subdural)
Intraoperative/postoperative hyperthermia
Dural tear
Cerebrospinal fluid leak
Meningitis
Postoperative mortality: 2.6%
Postoperative morbidity: 12%

Table 5.
Surgical complications associated with surgical treatment of craniosynostosis.

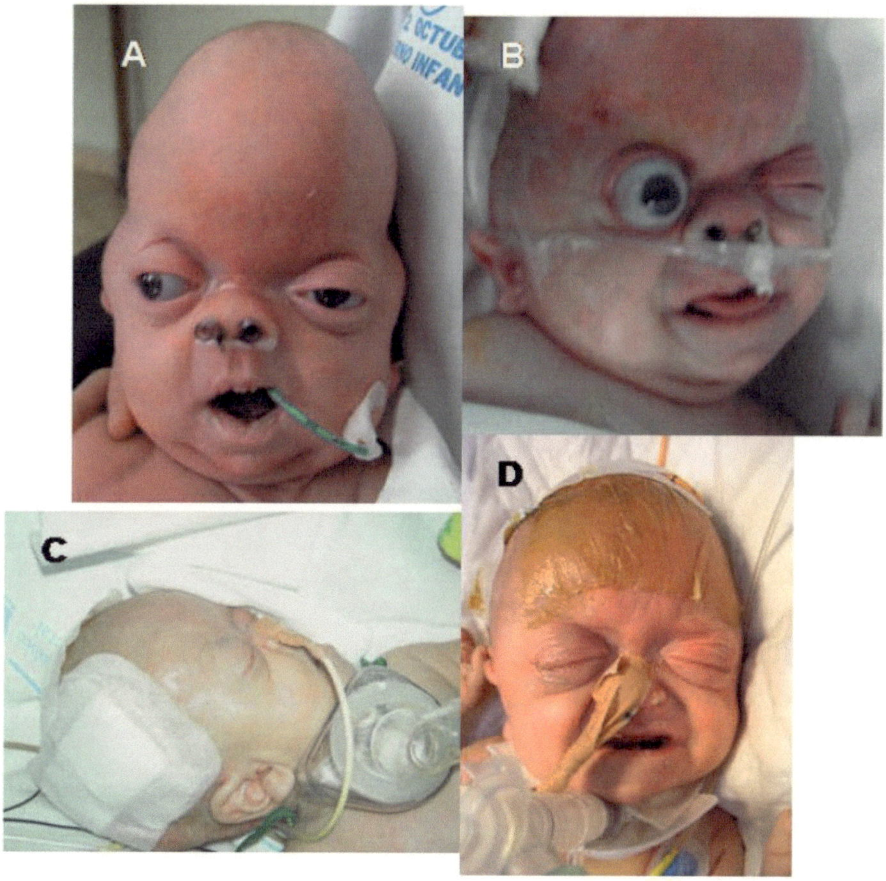

Figure 5.
3 month old with Pfeiffer syndrome. Cloverleaf skull [A]. GLobe herniation on Valsalva maneuver [B]. Post Op following fronto-facial distraction [C] [D]. Unfortunately, the patient died 18 months later due to infection related to tracheostomy [13].

than the actual procedure itself. The most common complications involved post-operative hyperthermia (13.43%) and cranial infection (7.3%). Other less frequent complications included CSF leaking, dura tears, and hematomas. Relapses occured in 11.56% of their cases which is a similar figure reported in other case studies. There is a significantly higher infection rate associated with relapse patients. Overall, 85% of their patients had successful outcomes, while negatively reported outcomes associated with those patients who had craniofacial syndromes. **Figure 5** portrays a case of a patient with Pfieffer syndrome who unfortunately died due to postoperative infection from the tracheostomy performed [13].

4. Conclusion

As craniosynostosis is a disorder that affects the development of the skull, the entire face is negatively impacted, which is evidenced by the treatment plan and treatment length that patients must face. The diagnostic and surgical approaches that we can take in order to remedy this disorder are wide and varied such as the joint surgical orthodontic approach. Overall, it is important to recognize the diagnostic features associated with craniosynostosis in order to plan the patient for the optimal form of care. While mortality is low, all the various craniosynostosis surgical techniques offer a wide range of complications that need to be understood and managed by the operator. Regular post-operative and long term followup can help ensure success of the operation.

Conflict of interest

The authors declare no conflict of interest.

Author details

Robert Pellecchia[1*], Kambiz Vatandoost[2], Anirudh Nair[2], Farajollah Soleimanzadeh[2], Benjamin Richardson[2] and Gunanand D. Persaud III[3]

1 Dentistry and Oral and Maxillofacial Surgery, Oral and Maxillofacial Surgery, New York, USA

2 Oral and Maxillofacial Surgery, New York, USA

3 Ramapo College, New York, USA

*Address all correspondence to: rpelloms@gmail.com

References

[1] Kajdic N, Spazzapan P, Velnar T. Craniosynostosis - recognition, clinical characteristics, and treatment. Bosnian Journal of Basic Medical Sciences. 2018;**18**(2):110-116. DOI: 10.17305/bjbms.2017.2083

[2] Mathijssen IM. Guideline for Care of Patients with the diagnoses of Craniosynostosis: Working group on Craniosynostosis. The Journal of Craniofacial Surgery. 2015;**26**(6):1735-1807. DOI: 10.1097/SCS.0000000000002016

[3] Barone CM, Jimenez DF. Endoscopic craniectomy for early correction of craniosynostosis. Plastic and Reconstructive Surgery. 1999;**104**(7):1965-1973; discussion 1974-5. DOI: 10.1097/00006534-199912000-00003

[4] Whitsell N, Meyer L. Craniosynostosis - a review for providers. South Dakota Medicine. 2021;**74**(2):83-88

[5] Looman WS, Kack Flannery AB. Continuing education evidence-based Care of the Child with Deformational Plagiocephaly, part I: Assessment and diagnosis. Journal of Pediatric Health Care. 2012;**26**:242-250

[6] Mulliken JB, Vander Woude DL, Hansen M, LaBrie RA, Scott RM. Analysis of posterior plagiocephaly: Deformational versus synostotic. Plastic and Reconstructive Surgery. 1999;**103**(2):371-380. DOI: 10.1097/00006534-199902000-00003

[7] Betances EM, Mendez MD, Das MJ. Craniosynostosis. Treasure Island (FL): StatPearls Publishing; 2022. p. 2022

[8] Staffenberg DA, Diaz-Siso JR, Flore RL. Fronto-orbital advancement: Description of surgical technique to complement the procedural cognition simulation in the craniofacial interactive virtual assistant-professional edition. The Journal of Craniofacial Surgery. 2019;**30**(2):473-477. DOI: 10.1097/SCS.0000000000005141

[9] Chong S, Wang KC, Phi JH, Lee JY, Kim SK. Minimally invasive Suturectomy and postoperative helmet therapy: Advantages and limitations. Journal of Korean Neurosurgical Association. 2016;**59**(3):227-232. DOI: 10.3340/jkns.2016.59.3.227

[10] Di Rocco F, Usami K, Protzenko T, et al. Results and limits of posterior cranial vault expansion by osteotomy and internal distractors. Surgical Neurology International. 2018;**9**:217

[11] Salokorpi N, Vuollo V, Sinikumpu JJ, Satanin L, Nestal Zibo H, Ylikontiola LP, et al. Increases in cranial volume with posterior cranial vault distraction in 31 consecutive cases. Neurosurgery. 2017;**81**:803-811

[12] Azoulay-Avinoam S, Bruun R, MacLaine J, Allareddy V, Resnick CM, Padwa BL. An overview of Craniosynostosis craniofacial syndromes for combined orthodontic and surgical management. Oral and Maxillofacial Surgery Clinics of North America. 2020;**32**(2):233-247. DOI: 10.1016/j.coms.2020.01.004

[13] Esparza J, Hinojosa J, García-Recuero I, Romance A, Pascual B, Martínez de Aragón A. Surgical treatment of isolated and syndromic craniosynostosis. Results and complications in 283 consecutive cases. Neurocirugía. 2008;**19**(6):509-529. DOI: 10.1016/s1130-1473(08)70201-x

[14] Kalmar CL, Swanson JW, Shakir S, et al. Spring-mediated cranioplasty for sagittal craniosynostosis. Neurosurgical Focus: Video FOCVID. 2021;**4**(2):V6. DOI: 10.3171/2021.1.FOCVID2060

Chapter 6

Assessment of Psychosocial Functioning among Patients with Cleft Lip/Palate and Their Mothers

Şeyma Akçay Gülşen, Belma Işik Aslan and Şadiye Bacık-Tırank

Abstract

The psychosocial functioning of children and adolescents with cleft lip and/or palate (CL/P) and their mothers was evaluated using a cross-sectional survey. The quality of life, depression, and self-esteem questionnaires were administered to CL/P patients and their mothers. The study included 69 individuals with CL/P between the ages of 6 and 18 and their mothers. According to the patient's age, CL/P patients and their mothers were divided into two groups: the infant group (6–12 years) and the adolescent group (13–18 years). Patients and mothers were requested to complete the questionnaires about life quality, self-esteem, and depression. According to the norm values of the Coopersmith Self-Esteem Scale, both child and adolescent groups have low self-esteem. However, adolescents' self-esteem levels were substantially lower than those of children ($p < 0.05$). There were no significant disparities between mothers of children and adolescents in terms of quality of life and self-esteem. The Beck depression scale scores of mothers of children were found to be greater than those of pubescent mothers ($p < 0.05$). Patients with CL/P tend to have lower self-esteem as they age; adolescents tend to have lower self-esteem than toddlers. In contrast, mothers of children with CL/P are less susceptible to melancholy than mothers of children.

Keywords: cleft lip/palate, psychosocial functioning, quality of life, depression, self-esteem

1. Introduction

Cleft lip and palate (CL/P) is a common congenital deformity causing upper lip, nose and alveolar malformation, esthetic and dental problems and functional disorders [1]. Modern interdisciplinary care for CL/P individuals aims at physical, functional and psychological rehabilitation [2]. Facial appearance has important effects on psychological well-being and communication skills [3].

Age is a crucial factor in the psychosocial development of individuals with cleft lip and palate (CL/P) and their mothers. Several studies suggest that the age of the patient may have an impact on their self-esteem, learning abilities and emotional well-being. For instance, Sischo et al. [4] found that older children with CL/P tend to have lower self-esteem than younger children, while Marques et al. [5]reported that mothers of younger children with CL/P experience higher levels of anxiety and depression compared to mothers of older children.

Speech-language problems and facial differences in CL/P patients can cause social reactions [6, 7], mocking and stigmatization [8] which may result in negative behavioral responses [9], low self-esteem, self-confidence and low quality of social interactions [3, 10, 11]. Age factor may affect the psychological development process in patients with CL/P. It was reported that adolescents with CL/P tend to have higher levels of self-esteem and lower levels of social anxiety and distress than adults [12]. Children and young adults with CL/P had greater behavioral problems and increased depression symptoms compared to healthy ones [13].

Cleft type also affects self-perception. The self-esteem of the individuals with cleft lip and palate (87%) was more affected than those with only cleft palate (75%), as the deformity in individuals with only cleft palate cannot be seen by others [14]. Despite some contradictory findings, the literature suggests that the relationship between age and psychosocial functioning in CL/P patients and their families is complex and multifaceted, influenced by factors such as the severity of the cleft, the timing of surgical interventions, and the presence of comorbidities. Nonetheless, to date, there have been limited studies investigating the psychosocial status of both individuals with CL/P and their mothers in a large-scale and multidimensional manner. Therefore, it is important to conduct further research to better understand the role of age in the psychosocial development of individuals with CL/P and their families.

2. Anxiety and depression in individuals with cleft lip and/or palate

Social anxiety is the state of anxiety that occurs when one is evaluated by others and worries about their perceptions. Physical appearance was found to be associated with social anxiety [15]. Individuals with CL/P and craniofacial anomalies are more prone to chronic social anxiety than unaffected ones [16]. Zeytinoğlu and Davey [17] reported that children born with CL/P tend to spend more time alone, have more negative interactions with their peers and participate in group games less frequently. These children with high levels of anxiety tend to exhibit more depressive behavior, especially outside the home and experience more bullying by their peers. Broder and Strauss [12] reported that 56% of individuals with cleft lip and palate, 49% of those with cleft palate and 33% of those with cleft lip need psychosocial support. It was reported that positive peer support in these individuals alleviated the negative effects of stigmatization [18].

3. Parents and mothers of individuals with CL/P

Situations that trigger or increase the stress of a family exponentially occur as a result of genetic or teratogenic factors that cause structural, functional, esthetic and psychological problems in children [19].

It was reported that mothers' first reactions to their babies born with CL/P are often shock, grief, insecurity, fear and guilt [20]. Fear of possible mental disorders in children is extremely common among parents [21]. This first effect of the child on his/her parents often persists for a long time [22]. However, cognitive and psychological damages of parents' intense stress reactions can be minimized by appropriate guidance and information shortly after birth [19].

Baby with CLP causes more trauma on their parents compared to ones with only cleft palate [21]. Turner et al. [3] considered that some of the parents had lower self-confidence due to CL/P. The process of lip repair can be an important determinant of mother-child attachment quality [17].

The purpose of present study is to asses psychosocial functioning among patients and mothers of these patients with CL/P by applying quality of life, depression and self-esteem surveys.

4. Methods

This study included 69 patients (32 females, 37 males) who applied to Gazi University Faculty of Dentistry Department of Orthodontics with CL/P and their mothers' participation. In order to conduct the study, the ethics committee approval dated 09.05.2017 and numbered 77,082,166-604.01.02 was obtained from Gazi University Ethics Committee.

Exclusion criteria for the study:

- patients with any mental problems that would prevent their ability to understand/answer questions or give scores,
- patients with different racial and ethnic backgrounds,
- patients with syndrome, and
- illiterate individuals aged 0–5 years.

Inclusion criteria for the study:

Individuals with CL/P aged 6–18 years and their mothers participated in the study voluntarily. The mean age of individuals with CL/P was 14 ± 3.9 years. Patients were divided into two groups as children and adolescents. Twenty-nine patients between the ages of 6 and 12 (mean age 9 ± 1.8 years) were included in the children group, and 40 patients between the ages of 13–18 (mean age 16.3 ± 1.7 years) were included in the adolescent group. Also, mothers of these patients were divided into two groups as mothers of children and mothers of adolescents. The purpose and content of the study were explained to the volunteer individuals and their mothers in detail and the surveys related to the study were asked to be answered individually.

As a data collection tool, a total of six surveys, three for patients with CL/P and three for their mothers were used. Also, additional questions were asked to the mothers in order to obtain sociodemographic descriptive information. The following surveys were applied to the patients with CL/P:

- Generic Health-Related Quality of Life Questionnaire for Children (Kid-KINDL) [23],
- Coopersmith Self-Esteem Inventory,
- Depression Scale for Children.

The Kid-KINDL scale (KINDer Lebensqualitätsfragebogen: Children Quality of Life Questionnaire) developed by Ravens-Sieberer and Bullinger [24], which consisted of 24 items and six subdimensions (physical well-being, emotional well-being, self-esteem, family, friends and school) was used to evaluate the generic quality of life in children. The scores obtained from the scale vary between 0 and 100. The scale does not have any cut-off point, and high scores indicate good quality of life [25]. There are three versions of the KINDL scale, which are based on self-report used in different age groups. These include Kiddy-KINDL for children aged 4–7 (version implemented via interviewer), Kid-KINDL for children aged 8–11 and Kiddo-KINDL for adolescents aged 12–16 [24]. In this study, Kid-KINDL scale was applied for the children group and Kiddo-KINDL version was used for the adolescent group.

The Coopersmith Self-Esteem Inventory is available in three versions: school form (8–15 years), adult form (16 years and older) and short form. The original forms, the school form and the adult form, consist of 58 items and the short form consists of 25 items. Fifty of the items are related to self-esteem and eight of them are related to lie scale; false items are used to measure the defensive attitude of individuals [26, 27]. The original form of this scale consisting of 58 items was used in our study. In the scale, items showing high self-esteem have a score of two and items showing low self-esteem have a score of 0. The scores that can be obtained from the scale vary between 0 and 100. In this scale, a score below 50 indicates a low self-esteem level while a score above 50 is considered as high self-esteem level [28].

In this study, 'the Depression Scale for Children' developed by Kovacs [29] was used to measure the depression scores of children. This is a self-assessment scale consisting of 27 items that can be applied to children aged 6–17 years. Each item receives 0, 1 or 2 points depending on the severity of the symptom. The reverse items in the scale are scored reversely. The maximum score is 54. The higher the score, the more severe depression [30]. The cut-off score is suggested as 19 [29, 31]. Those with a scale score of 19 or higher were considered pathological [32].

Three surveys were applied to the mothers:

- SF-36 Quality of Life Scale,
- Rosenberg Self-Esteem Scale,
- Beck Depression Inventory.

The SF-36 Quality of Life Scale is a 36-item test that the individual answers by himself/herself in order to obtain information about the general health status of the individual.

In the present study, "The Rosenberg Self-Esteem Scale" developed by Morris Rosenberg [33] was used to assess the self-esteem levels of mothers of patients with CL/P. The Rosenberg Self-Esteem Scale consists of 12 subscales. However, while the first subscale aimed to measure self-esteem directly, the other subscales were designed to measure situations thought to be related to self-esteem [34]. In the reliability and validity study conducted by Korkmaz [34] for the adaptation of the Rosenberg Self-Esteem Scale to adult individuals, the mean values of women for the 12 subunits of the scale were reported.

"The Beck Depression Scale" was used to assess the depression levels of mothers of patients with CL/P. This is a 21-item self-assessment scale which measures the symptoms of characteristic attitude and the cognitive, emotional and motivational tendencies in depression [35]. The scores to be obtained from the scale range from 0 to 63 and scores of 17 and above indicate the presence of depression [36].

4.1 Statistical analyses

Statistical analysis were performed using the IBM-SPSS (International Business Machines—Software Package for Social Sciences) Statistics software (version 23.0; IBM, Armonk, NY, USA). Comparison of cleft types and age, education and income levels of mothers between groups were performed using Chi-Square analysis. Mann–Whitney U test was used for comparisons between the groups. Pearson correlation analysis was performed to determine the relationship between the D1-self-esteem subscale and other subscales of the Rosenberg Self-Esteem Scale. P-value <0.05 was considered statistically significant.

5. Results

A total of 69 CL/P patients, including 15 females (51.7%) and 14 males (48.3%) in the children group and 17 females (42.5%) and 23 males (57.5%) in the adolescent group participated in the study. Gender distribution in groups and sociodemographic data distributions of these mothers are shown in **Table 1**.

Individuals with CL/P were between 6 and 18 years of age and their mean age was 13.3 ± 3.9 years. The children group was between 6 and 12 years of age (mean age: 9.2 ± 1.8 years). The adolescent group was between 13 and 18 years of age (mean age: 16.3 ± 1.7 years).

According to the sociodemographic data given in **Table 1**, the marital status of two individuals in the mothers of children group and five individuals in the mothers of adolescents were single.

When the age groups of the mothers of children were examined, it was seen that 37.9% of the mothers were between 25 and 34 years of age, 55.2% were between 35 and 44 years of age, and 6.9% were between 45 and 54 years of age. In the mothers of

		mother of child		**mother of adolescent**		**Total**		
Variable		n	%	n	%	n	%	p-value
Age	Under 25	0	0	1	2.5	1	1.4	0.012*
	Between 25 and 34	11	37.9	4	10	15	21.7	
	Between 35 and 44	16	55.2	24	60	40	58	
	Between 45 and 54	2	6.9	11	27.5	13	18.8	
	Total	29	100	40	100	69	100	
Gender of patients	Female	15	51.7	17	42.5	32	46.4	—
	Male	14	48.3	23	57.5	37	53.6	
Education Status	High school	26	89.7	36	90	62	89.9	0.701
	College	1	3.4	2	5	3	4.3	
	University	2	6.9	2	5	4	5.8	
	Total	29	100	40	100	69	100	

		mother of child		mother of adolescent		Total		
Marital status	Married	27	93.1	35	87.5	62	89.9	—
	Single	2	6.9	5	12.5	7	10.1	
	Total	29	100	40	100	69	100	
Income Level	1000–2000	18	62.1	10	25	28	40.6	0.083
	2000–3000	6	20.7	25	62.5	31	44.9	
	3000–4000	4	13.8	4	10	8	11.6	
	5000 and more	1	3.4	1	2.5	2	2.9	
	Total	29	100	40	100	69	100	
Are you responsible for other seriously ill patients in family?	Yes	0	0	2	5	2	2.9	—
	No	29	100	38	95	67	97.1	
	Total	29	100	40	100	69	100	
Can you mark your child's cleft type?	Only cleft lip	5	17.2	0	0	5	7.2	0.041*
	Only cleft palate	2	6.9	6	15	8	11.6	
	Unilateral CLP	17	58.6	25	62.5	42	60.9	
	Bilateral CLP	5	17.2	9	22.5	14	20.3	
	Total	29	100	40	100	69	100	
Does your child have any other illnesses	Yes	0	0	0	0	0	0	—
	No	29	100	40	100	69	100	
	Total	29	100	40	100	69	100	

**significant at the level 0.05.*

Table 1.
Gender and sociodemographic data distribution in groups.

adolescents group, 10% of the mothers were in the 25–34 age range, 60% were in the 35–44 age range, and 27.5% were in the 45–54 age range.

89.9% of the mothers are high school graduates, 5.8% are university graduates, and 4.3% are college graduates. In addition, 89.7% of the mothers of children and 90% of the mothers of adolescents are high school graduates.

While 40.6% of the families have income levels between 1000 and 2000 TL (Turkish lira), 44.9% between 2000 and 3000 TL, 11.6% between 3000 and 4000 TL, 2.9% have income levels of 5000 and above. While 62.1% of the families of children are in the 1000–2000 TL income group, 62.5% of the families of adolescents are in the 2000–3000 TL income group.

These mothers had no other serious patients to care for in the family.

While 11.6% of individuals with CL/P had only cleft palate, 60.9% had unilateral cleft lip and palate, 20.3% had bilateral cleft lip and palate cleft. While only cleft lip is seen in 17.2% of children group, it is not seen in the adolescent group.

According to the Chi-Square analysis, there was no significant difference between the groups of children and adolescents in terms of age, education level and income level ($p > 0.05$). There was a significant difference between the groups in terms of cleft types ($p < 0.05$). It is seen that the difference determined is due to only cleft lip and only cleft palate. While only cleft lip is seen at a higher rate in children, only cleft palate is seen at a higher rate in adolescents. Other cleft types were similar in adolescent and children groups.

6. Results of generic health-related quality of life questionnaire for children (kid-KINDL) assessment

There was no significant difference between the groups in terms of physical and emotional well-being, self-esteem, family, friends, school and total quality of life scores ($p > 0.05$). Although it was not statistically significant, it was observed that the scores of all subunits and total quality of life were higher in the children group (**Table 2**). Values in all units were within normal values for Turkish society.

Variable	Group	n	Mean	Median	Minimum	Maximum	SD	p-value
Bodily well-being	Child	29	16.0	16.0	9.0	20.0	2.8	0.512
	Adolescent	40	15.7	15.0	10.0	20.0	2.7	
	Total	69	15.8	16.0	9.0	20.0	2.7	
Emotional well-being	Child	29	16.2	17.0	9.0	20.0	2.6	0.316
	Adolescent	40	15.5	17.0	7.0	20.0	3.1	
	Total	69	15.8	17.0	7.0	20.0	2.9	
Self-respect	Child	29	13.9	14.0	6.0	20.0	4.0	0.487
	Adolescent	40	13.3	14.0	6.0	20.0	3.7	
	Total	69	13.6	14.0	6.0	20.0	3.8	
Family	Child	29	17.9	18.0	14.0	20.0	1.9	0.951
	Adolescent	40	18.6	18.0	11.0	65.0	8.0	
	Total	69	18.3	18.0	11.0	65.0	6.2	
Friend	Child	29	16.3	16.0	12.0	20.0	2.3	0.248
	Adolescent	40	15.5	16.0	10.0	20.0	2.4	
	Total	69	15.9	16.0	10.0	20.0	2.4	
School	Child	29	14.3	14.0	8.0	20.0	3.0	0.059
	Adolescent	40	13.0	14.0	8.0	16.0	2.1	
	Total	69	13.5	14.0	8.0	20.0	2.6	
Total Quality of Life	Child	29	94.6	96.0	77.0	115.0	10.4	0.197
	Adolescent	40	91.6	91.0	66.0	141.0	12.5	
	Total	69	92.8	92.0	66.0	141.0	11.7	

SD standard deviation.

Table 2.
Comparison of the mean values of generic health-related quality of life (QL) scale (Kid_KINDL) findings between child and adolescent groups.

6.1 Results of the Coopersmith self-esteem inventory and the depression scale for children assessments

In the Coopersmith Self-Esteem Inventory, self-esteem level below a score of 50 is considered low, and self-esteem level above a score of 50 is considered high [28]. According to this data, in this study, it was found that self-esteem level was low in children and adolescent groups with CL/P. When the individuals with CL/P were compared, it was seen that the self-esteem level of the adolescent group was significantly lower than the children group ($p < 0.05$) (**Table 3**).

In the Depression Scale for Children, those with a scale score of 19 or higher were considered pathological [32]. According to this data, the scale scores of children and adolescent groups with CL/P did not show any pathology in terms of depression. There was no significant difference between children and adolescent groups in terms of depression scores ($p > 0.05$) (**Table 4**).

Parameter	Group	n	Mean	Median	Minimum	Maximum	SD	p-value
Coopersmith Self-Esteem Scale	Child	29	28.0	29.0	0.0	39.0	6.7	0.006*
	Adolescent	40	25.8	25.0	19.0	34.0	3.5	
	Total	69	26.8	26.0	0.0	39.0	5.2	
Children's Depression Scale	Child	29	10.8	9.0	3.0	27.0	6.7	0.221
	Adolescent	40	8.6	7.0	2.0	21.0	5.0	
	Total	69	9.5	8.0	2.0	27.0	5.9	

**significant at the 0.05 level; SD standard deviation.*

Table 3.
Comparison of mean values of Coopersmith self-esteem and children's depression scale findings between child and adolescent groups.

Value of Depression	Mother of Child		Mother of Adolescent		Total	
	n	%	n	%	n	%
0–9 (Normal)	5	17.2	14	35	19	27.5
10–18 (mild-depression)	5	17.2	8	20	13	18.8
19–29 (moderate depression)	14	48.3	16	40	30	43.5
30–63 (severe depression)	5	17.2	2	5	7	10.1
Total	29	100	40	100	69	100
				Beck Depression Value		
Group	N	Mean	Median	Min-Max	SD	p-value
Mother of Child	29	21.41	22	2.00–43.00	10.82	0.032*
Mother of Adolescent	40	15.28	15.5	0.00	9.47	
Total	69	17.86	20	0	10.44	

**significant at the 0.05 level; SD standard deviation; Min minimum; Max Maximum.*

Table 4.
Distrubution of Beck depression scale findings and comparison of the mean values of Beck depression findings between mothers of child and adolescent groups.

6.2 Results regarding the assessment of Beck depression inventory applied to mothers

The mothers of children were found to have mostly moderate depression. Mild and severe depression rates were equal in this group. Mild depression rates were higher in the mothers of adolescents compared to the mothers of children (**Table 4**). According to Beck Depression Inventory scores, Beck Depression Inventory scores were significantly higher in the mothers of children than the mothers of adolescents. ($p < 0.05$) This finding indicates that the mothers of children are more prone to depression (**Table 4**).

6.3 Results regarding the assessment of SF-36 quality of life scale applied to mothers

There was no significant difference between the groups in terms of the scores in the SF-36 Quality of Life scale. ($p > 0.05$) (**Table 5**). In the study of Aydemir et al. [37], when the SF 36 community standard values were compared with the findings in this study, it was seen that the "Emotional Role Difficulty" and "Social Functioning" scores were below the average of the social standards in both groups.

Variable	Groups	n	Mean	Median	Minimum	Maximum	SD	p-value
Physical Function	Mother of Child	29	75.52	80	25	100	22.21	0.396
	Mother of Adolescent	40	73.13	80	15	100	20.65	
	Total	69	74.13	80	15	100	21.2	
Physical Role Difficulty	Mother of Child	29	68.1	75	0	100	31.97	0.321
	Mother of Adolescent	40	75.63	75	0	100	29.14	
	Total	69	72.46	75	0	100	30.36	
Emotional Role Difficulty	Mother of Child	29	68.97	66.67	0	100	36.66	0.979
	Mother of Adolescent	40	70.83	66.67	0	100	32.19	
	Total	69	70.05	66.67	0	100	33.89	
Energy/ Vitality	Mother of Child	29	57.59	55	25	90	17.81	0.771
	Mother of Adolescent	40	56.25	55	20	90	18.04	
	Total	69	56.81	55	20	90	17.82	
Mental Health	Mother of Child	29	69.1	72	32	100	20.42	0.798
	Mother of Adolescent	40	70.5	68	44	96	15.18	
	Total	69	69.91	68	32	100	17.44	

Variable	Groups	n	Mean	Median	Minimum	Maximum	SD	p-value
Social Functionality	Mother of Child	29	67.24	75	12.5	100	22.51	0.604
	Mother of Adolescent	40	70	75	12.5	100	23.31	
	Total	69	68.84	75	12.5	100	22.85	
Pain	Mother of Child	29	68.02	67.5	0	100	24.43	0.451
	Mother of Adolescent	40	71.94	77.5	10	100	21.16	
	Total	69	70.29	67.5	0	100	22.5	
General Health	Mother of Child	29	60.63	58.33	29.17	87.5	16.8	0.421
	Mother of Adolescent	40	57.08	58.33	20.83	87.5	14.71	
	Total	69	58.57	58.33	20.83	87.5	15.6	

SD standard deviation.

Table 5.
Comparison of the mean values of SF 36 quality of life scale findings between mothers of child and adolescent groups.

6.4 Results regarding the assessment of Rosenberg self-esteem scale applied to mothers

According to the results of the Rosenberg Self-Esteem Scale in **Table 6** and the comparison between the groups, no significant difference was observed between the groups of the mothers of children and adolescents ($p > 0.05$). Except for the subscales of D3 – Trust in people, D4 – Sensitivity to criticism, D6 – Fancifulness, it was seen that the mothers of children obtained higher scores than the mothers of adolescents, but this difference was not statistically significant.

In this scale consisting of 12 sections, there was no significant difference between the groups, while the sections of D1 – Self-esteem, D2 – Self-concept continuity and D3 – Trust in people were found to be at a high level in both groups. Sensitivity to criticism (D4), depressive affect (D5) and fancifulness (D6) were found to be at a low level in both groups. Both groups had moderate psychosomatic symptoms (D7). Both groups were found to feel a low level of threat in their interpersonal relationships (D8) and their degree of participation in discussions (D9) was low. Parental interest (D10) levels were found to be high in both groups, while relationship with the father (D11) was found to be at a low level (**Table 6**). When the mean values of the Rosenberg Self-Esteem Scale and the values of this study were compared for the women given in **Table 6**, similar scores were found in all other subscales except the Relationship with the Father subscale (D11). According to the mean values of the women, the relationship with the father, which is the D11 subscale, was moderate, yet it was found that there was a low level of relationship in this study. Psychical isolation (D12) was found to be low in both groups.

According to the Pearson's correlation analysis between the D1 subscales and other subscales, Self-esteem (D1) and Depressive affect (D5) and Psychical isolation (D12) have a similar and low-level relationship. ($p < 0.05$) D1 and D12 scores increased as D1 scores increased. According to these findings, it was concluded that as self-esteem decreased, depressive affect and psychical isolation increased.

Variable	Group	n	Mean	Median	Min	Max	SD	p-value
Self-respect	Mother of Child	29	0.86	0.75	0	2.41	0.6	0.991
	Mother of Adoles.	40	0.83	0.75	0	2.25	0.56	
	Total	69	0.84	0.75	0	2.41	0.57	
Continuity of Self-Concept	Mother of Child	29	2.97	3	1	5	1.21	0.707
	Mother of Adoles.	40	2.83	3	0	5	1.2	
	Total	69	2.88	3	0	5	1.19	
Trust in People	Mother of Child	29	1.52	1	0	3	0.83	0.575
	Mother of Adoles.	40	1.65	1	0	3	0.83	
	Total	69	1.59	1	0	3	0.83	
Sensitivity to Criticism	Mother of Child	29	1.72	2	1	3	0.53	0.927
	Mother of Adoles.	40	1.73	2	1	2	0.45	
	Total	69	1.72	2	1	3	0.48	
Depressive Affect	Mother of Child	29	1.93	2	0	6	1.56	0.891
	Mother of Adoles.	40	1.83	2	0	4	1.2	
	Total	69	1.87	2	0	6	1.35	
Imagination	Mother of Child	29	0.45	0	0	3	0.78	
	Mother of Adoles.	40	0.5	0	0	4	0.93	0.994
	Total	69	0.48	0	0	4	0.87	
Psychosomatic Symptoms	Mother of Child	29	3.72	2	0	10	3.19	0.844
	Mother of Adoles.	40	3.4	3	0	10	2.66	
	Total	69	3.54	3	0	10	2.88	
F. Threats in Interpersonal Relationship	Mother of Child	29	1.69	2	0	3	1.04	0.098
	Mother of Adoles.	40	1.28	1.5	0	3	1.04	
	Total	69	1.45	2	0	3	1.05	
Degree of Participation in Discussions	Mother of Child	29	0.62	0	0	2	0.73	
	Mother of Adoles.	40	0.5	0	0	2	0.64	0.525
	Total	69	0.55	0	0	2	0.68	

Variable	Group	n	Mean	Median	Min	Max	SD	p-value
Parental Interest	Mother of Child	29	1.55	1	0	8	2.06	
	Mother of Adoles.	40	1.4	0.5	0	7	1.88	0.815
	Total	69	1.46	1	0	8	1.94	
Relationship with Father	Mother of Child	29	2	1	0	6	1.91	0.227
	Mother of Adoles.	40	1.33	1	0	5	1.27	
	Total	69	1.61	1	0	6	1.59	
Psychic Isolation	Mother of Child	29	0.41	0	0	2	0.57	
	Mother of Adoles.	40	0.48	0	0	2	0.72	0.961
	Total	69	0.45	0	0	2	0.65	

**significant at the 0.05 level; SD standard deviation; Min minimum; Max Maximum; Adoles. Adolescent.*

Table 6.
Comparison of mean values of Rosenberg self-esteem scale findings between mothers of child and adolescent groups.

7. Discussion

Cleft lip and palate (CL/P) is a common congenital anomaly that affects the structure of the lip and/or the roof of the mouth. The psychosocial implications of CL/P can be significant, and research has explored various aspects of the psychosocial development of individuals with CL/P and their families. However, the role of age in the psychosocial development of CL/P patients and their mothers is not fully understood.

The psychological and social effects of deformity in individuals with CL/P have been studied since the 1960s. Less self-esteem, difficulty in learning and tendency to be more depressed and anxious were found in individuals with CL/P [38]. In this study, three questionnaires were applied to individuals with CL/P and their mothers, and their quality of life, self-esteem and depression levels were examined psychosocially in three different aspects. To the best of our knowledge, there are no studies in the literature addressing the psychosocial status of individuals in a large scale and in several dimensions as in this study. In addition, a limited number of studies conducted in Turkish society examined the psychosocial status of either individual with CL/P or only their families [39, 40]. However, there are no previous studies examining both individuals with CL/P and their mothers. Therefore, this study aimed to include both individuals with CL/P and their mothers.

Several studies have suggested that psychosocial functioning may be influenced by age in CL/P patients and their mothers. For example, a study by Sischo et al. [4] found that older children with CL/P had poorer self-esteem than younger children. Similarly, a study by Marques et al. [5] found that mothers of younger children with CL/P had higher levels of anxiety and depression than mothers of older children. These findings suggest that age may play an important role in the psychosocial development of CL/P patients and their mothers. However, some studies have reported contradictory or inconclusive results regarding the relationship between age and psychosocial functioning in CL/P patients and their families. For instance, a study by Richman and Eliason [41] found no significant difference in self-esteem between younger and older adolescents with CL/P. Similarly, a study by O'Brien et al. [42] found no significant relationship between age and maternal anxiety or depression.

Overall, the literature suggests that the relationship between age and psychosocial functioning in CL/P patients and their mothers is complex and may be influenced by various factors, such as the severity of the cleft, the timing of surgical interventions, and the presence of comorbidities. Further research is needed to clarify the role of age in the psychosocial development of individuals with CL/P and their families.

8. Case selection

In this study, no significant socioeconomic differences were found between the two age groups. In the study of Clark et al. [43], the relationship between the prevalence of CL/P and socioeconomic status could not be revealed. There is limited data about this relationship; therefore, furthermore research would provide better knowledge.

In this study, individuals with CL/P were divided into two groups at different age ranges, but no gender differentiation was made between the individuals. In a survey conducted by Bos and Prahl [44] to evaluate the quality of life of individuals with CL/P, no significant difference was found between males and females in quality of life levels. However, in the sample group where the age range was determined to be 8–15 years, the quality of life and emotional well-being of individuals aged 12 years and over were found to be lower than those of younger age groups. This indicates that quality of life levels change with age [44].

According to the survey conducted by Al-Ghamdi et al. [45], almost half of the parents who care for individuals with CL/P have difficulty managing their homes. In addition, it was reported that 50% of the parents were depressed before the treatment of their children, yet after the treatment, most parents had improved depression levels and only 11.9% had the same depression level. Based on these data, individuals in our study were examined in two age groups, including the groups of children (6–12 years) and adolescents (13–18 years). Mothers were also included in the study because usually mothers take care of the children and spend more time with their children.

8.1 Generic health-related quality of life for children

In this study, no statistically significant difference was found between the groups in any dimension (physical well-being, emotional well-being, self-esteem, family, friends and school) of the KINDL questionnaire used to evaluate the quality of life of individuals with CL/P. Similarly, there was no significant difference between groups in total quality of life. Also, quality of life scores of individuals with CL/P were found to be close to the normal values determined for Turkish society. These positive results can be explained by the quality of the team caring for them and the ability of these individuals to accept and cope with their situation.

Similar to our study, Naros et al. [46] applied the age-specific KINDL scale to 134 participants (47.8% of whom were females) aged 4–18 to evaluate the quality of life of individuals with CL/P in their study. In this study, compared with the normative data of surprisingly healthy individuals, higher quality of life was found in individuals with CL/P. However, the low rate of return of the questionnaires submitted caused bias in the results. Considering this situation, it was concluded that the quality of life in individuals with CL/P was not significantly lower than in healthy children.

In a survey conducted by Rivaldo et al. [47] to evaluate the quality of life of 94 individuals with cleft lip and palate aged 12 years and over, lower quality of life scores were reported by women or older individuals [47].

In a survey conducted by Ward et al. [48], which was applied to 75 individuals with CL/P (with a mean age of 13 years) and their caregivers and control group consisting of 75 healthy individuals (with a mean age of 13.9 years), generic oral health-related quality of life scores of children with CL/P were significantly lower than those of the control group. In addition, the negative effects of the orofacial cleft on quality of life scores were reported to be higher in individuals between the ages of 15–18 compared to the younger individuals.

8.2 Coopersmith self-esteem inventory

The Coopersmith Self-Esteem Inventory (CSI) has become the most popular instrument for measuring self-esteem both in our country and in the world. The Turkish version of the inventory was found to be consistent with the original scale [49]. When the findings of the Coopersmith Self-Esteem Inventory were evaluated, low self-esteem levels were found in both groups according to norm values. At the same time, self-esteem scores in the adolescent group were found to be significantly lower than the children group. Individuals with CL/P may have difficulty in expressing themselves in school life and speaking in public compared to normal individuals. This may affect their self-esteem negatively. In adolescence, individuals' awareness about themselves increases and social and emotional relationships with the environment increase. Therefore, low self-esteem levels are an expected result in the adolescent group.

In a survey conducted by Noor and Musa [14] on 60 individuals (12–17 years of age) with CL/P and their parents, it was reported that individuals with CL/P were mocked for their speech, teeth and lip appearance. It was shown that this situation has a negative effect on self-esteem, with a similar result in our study. In addition, cleft patients aged 16–17 thought that their self-confidence was more affected by their condition than younger individuals as they mature toward adulthood at these ages and interactions with the opposite sex are compulsory for them. Parents of these individuals also reported that cleft lip and palate caused mockery and negatively affected their children's self-esteem. It was stated that the most important features for individuals and their parents were teeth, nose, lip and speech, respectively, in descending order of priority.

In their study, Andrade and Angerami [50] measured self-esteem levels of 608 adolescents (17–20 years of age), 235 of whom were individuals with CL/P and 373 of them were normal individuals. Similar to our study, it was demonstrated that adolescents with CL/P behave differently from normal individuals and have lower self-esteem scores.

In a study by Gussy and Kilpatrick [10] comparing 23 adolescents with CL/P and control groups, no significant difference was found between the self-concept of individuals with CL/P and control groups.

8.3 Depression scale for children

The Depression Scale for Children, which was prepared by Kovacs [29], is based on Beck Depression Inventory and includes questions related to childhood depression, specific school status and friendship. This scale is the most commonly used scale in childhood depression, of which psychometric properties have been investigated most [32]. According to the findings of this scale, no significant difference was found between the children and adolescents in terms of depression scores. The fact that depression scores in both groups are within normal values can be explained by the individuals' good adaptation to their condition.

In the study of Fadeyibi et al. [51], in order to investigate the psychosocial status of 116 individuals with CL/P under the age of 6 and between the ages of 6–12, the responses of CL/P patients were evaluated by their parents. It was shown that individuals with CL/P have a high level of anxiety, depression and deterioration in general well-being. In the 6–12 age group, the effects were reported to be higher.

In a survey conducted by Berk et al. [16] on 85 Chinese adult individuals with CL/P and 85 healthy individuals, it was demonstrated that adult individuals with CL/P had significantly higher social anxiety and lower self-esteem scores than the control group.

As a result of their meta-analytical study on adolescents and adults with CL/P (2276) in non-Anglo populations, Hutchinson et al. [52] indicated that males with CL/P are more prone to psychosocial problems than females, and adults are more prone to psychosocial problems compared to adolescents. In general, it was determined that individuals with CL/P show lower psychosocial development than normal individuals, regardless of age, gender or culture.

8.4 SF-36 quality of life scale applied to mothers

SF-36 [53], which was developed in order to evaluate the quality of life, is a short yet comprehensive, strong, general health questionnaire in terms of psychometric properties [54]. It is used to compare the effects of the disease and the benefits of different treatments in all age, disease and treatment groups. To date, it has been widely used in the general population [54]. Its reliability and validity study was conducted in Turkey [55]. When the subscales were evaluated, no statistically significant difference was found between the groups of the mothers of children and adolescents. In general, when the norm values of the SF-36 Scale for Turkish society were examined, all the remaining subscales were within the norm values except for the social functionality subscale in the mothers of children and adolescents with CL/P. Since the individuals with CL/P require almost lifelong multidisciplinary teamwork, families have to spend more time with their children, which leads to lower social activity and lower energy. Therefore it was an expected result that mothers' energy/vitality and related social functionality scores would be low.

In the study conducted by Aslan et al. [39], family functions and quality of life of the parents having children with CL/P were evaluated and compared with a normal group. In the study, parents were grouped according to the children's age ranges as 0–6, 7–12 and 13–18, and no significant differences were detected in the quality of life of parents between the CL/P and control groups in 0–6 and 7–12 age groups. However, it was reported that quality of life scores in physical, social and psychological fields was lower in the parents of adolescents with CL/P between the ages of 13–18 compared to the control group.

Antunes et al. [56] found that the quality of life of the families having children with CL/P (4–17 years) was negatively affected compared to the control group because they had to spend more time with their children. When the quality of life of the families of children with CL/P was compared according to the visibility of the deformity, the differences were found to be insignificant.

Crerand et al. [57] reported that stress factors such as the experience of having a child with CL/P could offer opportunities for the formation of protective factors that can improve families' resilience (for example, low levels of family conflict, healthy adjustment and expression).

In a study by Tobiasen and Hiebert [58], it was found that parents of the children with CL/P were significantly more tolerant toward behavioral problems in their children compared to parents of normal children. This result revealed that families having children with CL/P develop strategies to solve problems since they face many problems and stresses from the birth of their children.

In the pilot study by Eiserman [59], it was reported that parents of children with CL/P had positive outcomes such as empathy and increased sensitivity to others, ability to help, closer relationships and acceptance of life challenges, improved communication skills and greater adaptation.

In a study conducted by Baker et al. [60] in order to examine the coping strategies and psychological discomfort levels of 103 families having children with CL/P, the parents were divided into three groups according to the age range of their children (0–6 years, 7–12 years and 13–18 years). It was demonstrated that families with young children were affected more depending on age. This situation was explained by the necessity of more comprehensive treatment, more frequent surgical intervention and clinical visits at younger ages.

8.5 Rosenberg self-esteem scale applied to mothers

In this study, self-esteem levels were high and depressive effect levels were low in both groups and no significant difference was found between the groups of the mothers of children and adolescents.

According to the results of the survey conducted by Weatherley-White et al. [61] on 52 families in India, 64% of the parents stated that their children's social interaction was not restricted and they were not ashamed of this situation, while 26% stated that they imposed some restrictions and 10% stated that they completely isolated their children from the society and did not allow them to go out of the house or go to school. The responses of the majority of the parents in this study are similar to the subscales of the high level of self-esteem (D1), low level of depressive effect (D5), high level of trust in people (D3) and low level of sensitivity to criticism (D4) in our study.

8.6 Beck depression inventory applied to mothers

The Beck Depression Inventory was found to be a reliable scale that can be applied in a short time, of which reliability and validity study was conducted in Turkey [62]. In this study, it was found that mothers of children were significantly more prone to depression than mothers of adolescents. It is an expected result as mothers of children with CL/P are more concerned with the care of their children and more frequent surgical intervention and physician control are required in individuals of this age.

We have not met any studies evaluating depression levels in children and adolescents with CL/P and/or their parents. In other studies regarding depression, stress levels of families of individuals with CL/P in prenatal or infancy period before or after surgery were evaluated.

In the study of Nelson et al. [63], anxiety, depression and perceived stress levels of parents having 12–24 months old babies with CL/P were evaluated. Authors reported that anxiety and perceived stress scale were significantly higher in parents who blamed themselves for this condition in their babies; however, depression scores were not significantly higher [63].

O'Hanlon et al. [64] investigated the effects of prenatal diagnosis of CL/P in their parents. According to the results, these parents were found to feel significantly more guilty compared to the parents in the control group.

In the study of Tabaquim and Marquesini [19], the stress levels of the mothers and fathers before surgery of CL/P patients were evaluated, and it was revealed that stress level was high in 21.4% of the parents, moderate in 28.6% and low in 50% before surgery. On the other hand, stress level was high in 7.1%, moderate in 21.4% and low in 71.4% of parents after surgery.

It is reported that parents are concerned about operations, physical appearance and social functionality [17]. Therefore parents should be informed about how to communicate with their children with CL/P and what types of surgeries and medical procedures they will undergo in the future [65].

8.7 Limitations of the study

In our study, the cleft type of patients was not classified because of the limited number of isolated palatal or lip cleft cases. Further studies with increased number of patients would be better to investigate the impact of the type of cleft on the psychosocial functioning of both patients and their parents. In addition, the mothers of individuals with CL/P should be compared with control group mothers. Finally, this study identifies the psychosocial functioning among patients with CL/P and their mothers at only one point of time study. Long-term evaluation will provide us better understanding of whether issues regarding psychosocial functioning change over time.

9. Conclusion

In this study, the following results were obtained:

There was no significant difference in terms of quality of life between the groups of children and adolescents with CL/P, and the mothers of children and adolescents. Quality of life levels were found to be close to the mean values for both individuals with CL/P and their mothers.

Low self-esteem levels were determined in both children and adolescents with CL/P. Self-esteem level of the adolescent group was significantly lower than the children group.

Self-esteem levels were not found to be significantly different between the mothers of children and the mothers of adolescents. High self-esteem levels were observed in both groups.

No significant difference was found between the children and adolescents in terms of depression scores.

Beck Depression Inventory scores were higher in the mothers of children than the mothers of adolescents. This result indicates that the mothers of children with CL/P are more prone to depression.

Psychosocial and behavioral problems may occur in children and adolescents with CL/P due to their deformities. In addition to treatment for the deformities and functions of individuals with CL/P, good psychological support is needed to improve their psychosocial status. In addition, healthy individuals should be informed appropriately in order to prevent situations such as mocking, bullying and stigmatization that cause psychosocial and behavioral problems and to change society's perspective and prejudice against these individuals with CL/P.

While each family needs to be evaluated within itself, mothers who take care of individuals with CL/P should be properly and thoroughly informed by the multidisciplinary team about the situation and care of their children. Appropriate psychosocial support is required to reduce stress and depression levels in mothers.

Acknowledgements

The authors would like to thank Prof. Dr. Ayşe Gülşen for their thoughtful suggestions regarding both the development of this project and revision of this manuscript. In addition, the authors would like to thank the participants and their families for their significant contribution to this study.

Declaration of conflicting interests

The author(s) declared no potential conflicts of interest with respect to the research, authorship and/or publication of this article.

Funding

The author(s) received no financial support for the research, authorship and/or publication of this article.

Supplemental material

Supplemental material for this article is available online.

Author details

Şeyma Akçay Gülşen[1], Belma Işik Aslan[2*] and Şadiye Bacık-Tırank[3]

1 Independent Researcher, Ankara, Turkey

2 Department of Orthodontics, Gazi University Dentistry Faculty, Ankara, Turkey

3 Faculty of Health Sciences, Department of Speech and Language Therapy, Gazi University, Ankara, Turkey

*Address all correspondence to: belmaslan2003@yahoo.com

References

[1] Fisher MD, Fisher DM, Marcus JR. Correction of the cleft nasal deformity: From infancy to maturity. Clinics in Plastic Surgery. 2014;**2**:283-299

[2] Warschausky S, Kay JB, Buchman S, Halberg A, Berger M. Health-related quality of life in children with craniofacial anomalies. Plastic And Reconstructive Surgery. 2002;**110**(2):409-414

[3] Turner SR, Thomas PWN, Dowell T, Rumsey N, Sandy JR. Psychological outcomes amongst cleft patients and their families. British Journal of Plastic Surgery. 1997;**50**(1):1-9

[4] Sischo L, Broder HL, Phillips C, Dillard J. Measuring psychological characteristics of young children with cleft lip and palate: A comparison of self-report and proxy ratings. The Cleft Palate-Craniofacial Journal. 2011;**48**(3):309-319

[5] Marques LS, Ramos-Jorge ML, Paiva SM, Pordeus IA, Malheiros AS. Anxiety and depression in parents of Brazilian children with cleft lip and/or palate. Journal of Clinical Pediatric Dentistry. 2015;**39**(5):432-436

[6] Kapp-Simon KA, Simon DJ, Kristovich S. Self-perception, social skills, adjustment, and inhibition in young adolescents with craniofacial anomalies. The Cleft Palate-Craniofacial Journal. 1992;**29**(4):352-356

[7] Millard T, Richman LC. Different cleft conditions, facial appearance, and speech: Relationship to psychological variables. The Cleft Palate-Craniofacial Journal. 2001;**38**(1):68-75

[8] Shaw WC, Meek SC, Jones DS. Nicknames, teasing, harassment and the salience of dental features among school children. British Journal of Orthodontics. 1980;**7**(2):75-80

[9] Pope AW, Ward J. Factors associated with peer social competence in preadolescents with craniofacial anomalies. Journal of Pediatric Psychology. 1997;**22**(4):455-469

[10] Gussy M, Kilpatrick N. The self-concept of adolescents with cleft lip and palate: A pilot study using a multidimensional/hierarchical measurement instrument. International Journal of Paediatric Dentistry. 2006;**16**(5):335-341

[11] Turner SR, Rumsey N, Sandy JR. Psychological aspects of cleft lip and palate. The European Journal of Orthodontics. 1998;**20**(4):407-415

[12] Broder H, Strauss R. Psychological problems and referrals among oral-facial team patients. Journal of Rehabilitation. 1991;**57**(1):31-36

[13] Hunt O, Burden D, Hepper P, Stevenson M, Johnston C. Self-reports of psychosocial functioning among children and young adults with cleft lip and palate. The Cleft Palate-Craniofacial Journal. 2006;**43**(5):598-605

[14] Noor SNFM, Musa S. Assessment of patients' level of satisfaction with cleft treatment using the cleft evaluation profile. The Cleft Palate-Craniofacial Journal. 2007;**44**(3):292-303

[15] Leary MR, Kowalski RM. Social Anxiety. New York: Guilford Press; 1995

[16] Berk NW, Cooper ME, Liu YE, Marazita ML. Social anxiety in Chinese adults with oral-facial clefts. The

Cleft Palate-Craniofacial Journal. 2001;**38**(2):126-133

[17] Zeytinoglu S, Davey MP. It's a privilege to smile: Impact of cleft lip palate on families. Families, Systems & Health. 2012;**30**(3):265-277

[18] Tiemens K, Nicholas D, Forrest CR. Living with difference: Experiences of adolescent girls with cleft lip and palate. The Cleft Palate-Craniofacial Journal. 2013;**50**(2):27-34

[19] Tabaquim MDLM, Marquesini MAM. Study of the stress of parents of patients with cleft lip and palate in a surgical process. Estudos de Psicologia (Campinas). 2013;**30**(4):517-524

[20] Ripley IL, Kallaus J, Mcdermott MM. The child with cleft lip palate. The American Journal of Nursing. 1965;**65**(4):124-127

[21] Tisza VB, Gumpertz E. The parents' reactıon to the bırth and early care of children with cleft palate. Pediatrics. 1962;**30**(1):86-90

[22] Moraes MCAF, Buffa MJMB, Motti TFG. As atividades expressivas e recreativas em crianças com fissura labiopalatina hospitalizadas: visão dos familiares. Revista Brasileira de Educação Especial. 2009;**15**(3):453-470

[23] Eser E, Yüksel H, Baydur H, Erhart M, Saatli G, Özyurt BC, et al. Çocuklar İçin Genel Amaçlı Sağlıkla İlgili Yaşam Kalitesi Ölçeği (Kid-KINDL) Türkçe Sürümünün Psikometrik Özellikleri. Turk Psikiyatri Dergisi. 2008;**19**(4):409-417

[24] Ravens-Sieberer U, Bullinger M. Assessing health-related quality of life in chronically ill children with the German KINDL: First psychometric and content analytical results. Quality of Life Research. 1998;**7**(5):399-407

[25] Ayfer EKİM, Ayşe FO. 8-12 yaş arası işitme engelli çocuklarda yaşam kalitesi. Ankara Sağlık Hizmetleri Dergisi. 2012;**11**(1):17-23

[26] Myhill J, Lorr M. The coopersmith self-esteem inventory: Analysis and partial validation of a modified adult form. Journal of Clinical Psychology. 1978;**34**(1):72-76

[27] Ryden MB. An adult version of the Coopersmith self-esteem inventory: Test-retest reliability and social desirability. Psychological Reports. 1978;**43**(3):1189-1190

[28] Tözün M. Benlik saygısı. Actual Medicine. 2010:52-57

[29] Kovacs M. Rating scales to assess depression in school-aged children. Acta Paedopsychiatrica: International Journal of Child & Adolescent Psychiatry. 1981;**46**(5-6):305-315

[30] Oy B. Cocuklar icin Depresyon Olcegi gecerlik ve guvenirlik calismasi. Turk Psikiyatri Dergisi. 1991;**2**:137-140

[31] Kovacs M. The children's depression inventory (CDI). Psychopharmacology Bulletin. 1985;**21**(4):995-998

[32] Aysev A, Ulukol B, Ceyhun G. Çalışan ve okuyan çocukların "çocuklar için depresyon ölçeği" ile değerlendirilmesi. Ankara Üniversitesi Tıp Fakültesi Mecmuası. 2000;**53**(01):27-30

[33] Rosenberg M. Society and the Adolescent Self-Image. Princeton, New Jersey: Princeton University Press; 1965

[34] Korkmaz M. Yetişkin örneklem için bir benlik saygısı ölçeğinin güvenirlik ve geçerlik çalışması. Yüksek Lisans Tezi, İzmir: Ege Üniversitesi, Sosyal Bilimler Enstitüsü; 1996

[35] Beck AT, Ward C, Mendelson M, Mock J, Erbaugh J. Beck depression inventory (BDI). Archives of General Psychiatry. 1961;**4**(6):561-571

[36] Hisli N. Beck Depresyon Envanterinin gecerliligi uzerine bit calisma (a study on the validity of Beck depression inventory). Psikoloji Dergisi. 1988;**6**:118-122

[37] Aydemir Ö, Ergün H, Soygür H, Kesebir S, Tulunay C. Major Depresif Bozuklukta Yaşam Kalitesi: Kesitsel Bir Çalışma. Türk Psikiyatri Dergisi. 2009;**20**(3):205-211

[38] Broder HL, Richman LC, Matheson PB. Learning disability, school achievement, and grade retention among children with cleft: A two-center study. The Cleft Palate- Craniofacial Journal. 1998;**35**(2):127-131

[39] Aslan BI, Gülsen A, Tirank SB, Findikçioglu K, Uzuner FD, Tutar H, et al. Family functions and life quality of parents of children with cleft lip and palate. Journal of Craniofacial Surgery. 2018;**29**(6):1614-1618

[40] Sokucu O, Nalcaci R, Ozturk F, Toy S. Dudak damak yarıklı bireylerin kendini- kabul düzeylerinin değerlendirilmesi. Cumhuriyet Dental Journal. 2011;**11**(1):35-39

[41] Richman LC, Eliason MJ. Self-esteem and craniofacial anomalies: A 15-year follow-up. Cleft Palate-Craniofacial Journal. 2008;**45**(1):33-37

[42] O'Brien K, Collett BR, Leroux B, Speltz ML, Squire JR, Edwards TC. Anxiety symptoms and disorders in adolescents with cleft lip and palate. Cleft Palate-Craniofacial Journal. 2009;**46**(4):386-392

[43] Clark JD, Mossey PA, Sharp L, Little J. Socioeconomic status and orofacial clefts in Scotland, 1989 to 1998. The Cleft Palate-Craniofacial Journal. 2003;**40**(5):481-485

[44] Bos A, Prahl C. Oral health–related quality of life in Dutch children with cleft lip and/ or palate. The Angle Orthodontist. 2011;**81**(5):865-871

[45] Al-Ghamd M, Bayoumi A, Zahran M. Quality of life of cleft lip and/or palate patients' caregivers in Jeddah. Journal of Dental and Oral Health. 2016;**2**(7):1-4

[46] Naros A, Brocks A, Kluba S, Reinert S, Krimmel M. Health-related quality of life in cleft lip and/or palate patients–a cross-sectional study from preschool age until adolescence. Journal of Cranio-Maxillofacial Surgery. 2018;**46**(10):1758-1763

[47] Rivaldo EG, Russomano RP, Vargas-Ferreira F, Pinto JHN, Frasca LCF. Impact of cleft lip and palate on oral health-related quality of life (OHRQOL) in Brazilian patients. Pesquisa Brasileira em Odontopediatria e Clinica Integrada. 2017;**17**(1):1-9

[48] Ward JA, Vig KW, Firestone AR, Mercado A, Da Fonseca M, Johnston W. Oral health–related quality of life in children with orofacial clefts. The Cleft Palate- Craniofacial Journal. 2013;**50**(2):174-181

[49] Güloğlu B, Aydın G. Coopersmith Özsaygı Envanteri'nin Faktör Yapısı. Eğitim ve Bilim. 2001;**26**(122):66-71

[50] Andrade DD, Angerami ELS. The self-esteem of adolescents with and without a cleft lip and/or palate. Revista Latino-Americana de Enfermagem. 2001;**9**(6):37-41

[51] Fadeyibi IO, Coker OA, Zacchariah MP, Fasawe A, Ademiluyi SA. Psychosocial effects of cleft lip and palate

on Nigerians: The Ikeja-Lagos experience. Journal of Plastic Surgery and Hand Surgery. 2012;**46**(1):13-18

[52] Hutchinson K, Wellman MA, Noe DA, Kahn A. The psychosocial effects of cleft lip and palate in non-Anglo populations: A cross-cultural meta-analysis. The Cleft Palate-Craniofacial Journal. 2011;**48**(5):497-508

[53] Ware JE Jr, Sherbourne CD. The MOS 36-item short-form health survey (SF-36). I. Conceptual framework and item selection. Medical Care. 1992;**30**(6):473-483

[54] Boueri FM, Bucher-Bartelson BL, Glenn KA, Make BJ. Quality of life measured with a generic instrument (short Form-36) improves following pulmonary rehabilitation in patients with COPD. Chest Journal. 2001;**119**(1):77-84

[55] Koçyiğit H, Aydemir O, Ölmez N, Memiş A. SF-36′ nin Türkçe için güvenilirliği ve geçerliliği. Ege Fizik Tedavi ve Rehabilitasyon Dergisi. 1999;**12**:102-106

[56] Antunes LS, Maués CPR, Nadaes MR, Costa MC, Küchler EC, Antunes LAA. The impact of nonsyndromic oral clefts on family quality of life. Special Care in Dentistry. 2014;**34**(3):138-143

[57] Crerand CE, Rosenberg J, Magee L, Stein MB, Wilson-Genderson M, Broder HL. Parent-reported family functioning among children with cleft lip/palate. The Cleft Palate-Craniofacial Journal. 2015;**52**(6):651-659

[58] Tobiasen JM, Hiebert JM. Parents' tolerance for the conduct problems of the child with cleft lip and palate. The Cleft Palate Journal. 1984;**21**(2):82-85

[59] Eiserman W. Unique outcomes and positive contributions associated with facial difference: Expanding research and practice. The Cleft Palate-Craniofacial Journal. 2001;**38**(3):236-244

[60] Baker SR, Owens J, Stern M, Willmot D. Coping strategies and social support in the family impact of cleft lip and palate and parents' adjustment and psychological distress. The Cleft Palate-Craniofacial Journal. 2009;**46**(3):229-236

[61] Weatherley-White RCA, Eiserman W, Beddoe M, Vanderberg R. Perceptions, expectations, and reactions to cleft lip and palate surgery in native populations: A pilot study in rural India. The Cleft Palate-Craniofacial Journal. 2005;**42**(5):560-564

[62] Aktürk Z, Dağdeviren N, Türe M, Tuğlu C. Birinci basamak için beck depresyon tarama ölçeği'nin Türkçe çevriminin geçerlik ve güvenirliği. Türkiye Aile Hekimliği Dergisi. 2005;**9**(3):117-122

[63] Nelson J, O'leary C, Weinman J. Causal attributions in parents of babies with a cleft lip and/or palate and their association with psychological well-being. The Cleft Palate- Craniofacial Journal. 2009;**46**(4):425-434

[64] O'hanlon K, Camic PM, Shearer J. Factors associated with parental adaptation to having a child with a cleft lip and/or palate: The impact of parental diagnosis. The Cleft Palate-Craniofacial Journal. 2012;**49**(6):718-729

[65] Frain MP, Lee GK, Berven NL, Tansey T, Tschopp MK, Chronister J. Use of resiliency model of family stress, adjustmentandadaptationbyrehabilitation counselors. Journal of Rehabilitation. 2007;**73**(3):18-25